Praise for

CODE GRAY

"Timely and nuanced, Farzon Nahvi's exploration of healthcare probes the grayscale of life, from the most human of details to the overarching systemic issues. As we grapple with unprecedented challenges to both healthcare and society, we are ever more in need of clear-eyed books like *Code Gray*."
—Danielle Ofri, MD, PhD, author of
When We Do Harm: A Doctor Confronts Medical Error

"A provocative and meaningful book, *Code Gray* takes us to the hard places in health care, where the 'correct' treatment choices can be impossible to know. Fortunately, Dr. Nahvi is caring and percipient. He is an amazing guide to the portal separating life and death, sickness and health, and the real world and the hospital—that is, the modern Emergency Department."
—Theresa Brown, *New York Times* bestselling author of
Healing: When A Nurse Becomes a Patient and *The Shift*

"At turns discomfiting and often bracing, the book uses one specific case (a previously healthy woman who has a heart attack) as a stalking horse to present [Nahvi's] real point, namely that when it comes to life and death, what we see and what we say are rarely black and white."
—*Bloomberg Businessweek*

"Farzon Nahvi creates a fast-moving primer in medical ethics and humanism while addressing many decisions made daily in the emergency room that are critical to life and well-being and always made with substantial uncertainty."

—Lewis R. Goldfrank,
Professor of Emergency Medicine,
New York University Grossman School of Medicine;
Attending Physician Bellevue Hospital Center

"A window into not only what happens in Emergency Departments and hospitals around the country but also into the intense feelings experienced by those involved. Dr. Nahvi expertly captures the humanity of caring for patients as well, the toll it takes on each of us and the machinations we desperately construct to survive. *Code Gray* is poignant and painful and an important read."

—Anand Swaminathan, MD, MPH,
Assistant Professor of Emergency Medicine,
Staten Island University Hospital/Northwell Health

"Compelling. . . . A transparent and thought-provoking account of the intense pressure, tragedy, ethical dilemmas, and uncertainty that ER doctors face in the course of their duties."

—*Washington Independent Review of Books*

CODE GRAY

Death, Life, and Uncertainty in the ER

FARZON A. NAHVI, M.D.

SIMON & SCHUSTER PAPERBACKS

New York   London   Toronto   Sydney   New Delhi

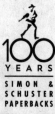

An Imprint of Simon & Schuster, Inc.
1230 Avenue of the Americas
New York, NY 10020

Copyright © 2023 by Farzon Nahvi, M.D.

All rights reserved, including the right to reproduce this book or portions
thereof in any form whatsoever. For information, address
Simon & Schuster Subsidiary Rights Department,
1230 Avenue of the Americas, New York, NY 10020.

First Simon & Schuster trade paperback edition February 2024

SIMON & SCHUSTER PAPERBACKS and colophon are
registered trademarks of Simon & Schuster, Inc.

Simon & Schuster: Celebrating 100 Years of Publishing in 2024

For information about special discounts for bulk purchases,
please contact Simon & Schuster Special Sales at
1-866-506-1949 or business@simonandschuster.com.

The Simon & Schuster Speakers Bureau can bring authors to your live event.
For more information or to book an event, contact the
Simon & Schuster Speakers Bureau at 1-866-248-3049
or visit our website at www.simonspeakers.com.

Interior design by Ruth Lee-Mui

1   3   5   7   9   10   8   6   4   2

Library of Congress Cataloging-in-Publication Data is available.

ISBN 978-1-9821-6029-6
ISBN 978-1-9821-6031-9 (pbk)
ISBN 978-1-9821-6032-6 (ebook)

For my wife, Vivian,
and my sister, Barin.

Contents

CONTENTS

Author's Note

Each person and scenario in this book is based on my memory of a real experience I have had in the emergency room. Nevertheless, descriptions of specific individuals have been altered. Names, ages, and other identifying characteristics such as gender, profession, geographic location, familial relationship, and medical history—even the description of a haircut or a tattoo—have been changed throughout this book. Any resemblance to persons living or dead resulting from these changes is entirely coincidental and unintentional.

THE NOVEL CORONAVIRUS

What follows is a series of text messages between a group of ER physicians across the country.

February 28, 2020

LA: So, crazy coronavirus story to get everyone worked up. Family of four presented with fever and cough after just returning from South Korea where a close family member they had contact with is hospitalized for coronavirus. Any guesses what the CDC recommended?

DE: My guess is no testing?

SE: I don't think I want to know.

KB: New guidelines say test

LA: Haha yea no testing

WS: Yes. They don't want to test anyone.
We have so many of those at my shop
Every time [we call the department of health] they say don't test.

BX: Best way you can say you don't have cases is by not looking for them.

CODE GRAY

March 2, 2020

WS: ███████ hospital has a Covid case

KB: A second Manhattan case?

WS: I think it's the first [test confirmed case]

SE: It's crazy to think NYC and LA aren't already full of it.
It's just that nobody is testing.

PROLOGUE

March 5, 2020

ES: ▮▮▮▮▮▮▮ hospital has one now [too]

KB: Has anyone tested for community spread? NYC Dept of Health only tests for known contacts or travel risk now.

QS: Yea, [we] haven't tested for community yet

BX: Seems dumb when you're potentially more likely to be exposed to it in NYC at this point

ES: That's my favorite part

HO: Astronaut applications on usajobs.gov open tomorrow for anyone interested in escaping Earth

CODE GRAY

March 11, 2020

ES: It's starting here
About to intubate for respiratory failure. Bilateral
interstitial pneumonia. Hypoxic failure.[1]
It's going to be a dumpster fire when there are
multiple

WS: ES that's almost certainly it. It's all over. ███████
hospital, ███████, ███████, my hospital

ES: Yeah

KB: Just intubated a confirmed corona.
My plan as of now is if you fail nasal cannula and need
a nonrebreather you are likely to progress rapidly and
I'm going to get ready to tube you[2]

DE: Same

WS: Seems better to just rapidly intubate. It's source
control.
Of course, we will run out of vents and ICU beds
but . . .

KB: That's my practice until we run out of vents[3]

PROLOGUE

March 20, 2020

KB: Just got off a phone call with our ventilator rationing committee.

QS: I just followed up on everyone I've admitted (and all age ranges and all without respiratory distress at time of admission but with other factors, whether it was hypoxia, or how bad chest X-ray was, or age etc.) and like 90% of them are now intubated

JJ: Wow that's insane—all Covid positive?

QS: Ya. And that's just my patients. I was just chart checking the ICU/Step Down Unit patients and similar story for most of them

WH: Miss you all . . . just got out of a crazy shift . . . everyone is pretty much positive now

KB: We aren't liberating any of our vented patients

• • •

"We aren't liberating any of our vented patients," my friend had written in his text message. His language was revealing. One does not require liberation from a savior, of course, but from an oppressor. And so, while the country was celebrating healthcare workers as heroes, we knew that the truth of our circumstance was much more complex.

We were scrambling to take action despite having no clear idea of what the right course of action was. We prescribed medications and performed interventions while wondering aloud whether they would do any good. Our lack of information did not preclude our mandate to act. And so, at best, our efforts were a paradox: we did what we could to save our patients from their disease, and then, later, we would do what we could to liberate them from those very efforts.

This is not unusual. As much as we may prefer a narrative where the right course of action is clear and where what is helpful shares no border with what may cause harm, such a narrative has never reflected the reality of my experience. An honest narrative is never a clean one. Like so many things in our lives, there was no playbook and no perfect solution. We existed, as we often do, within a series of impossible circumstances.

Reality is subtle, grayscale, and nuanced. It is playing the role of both savior and oppressor at the same time. It is taking action while recognizing that action to be imperfect, and moving forward despite being unable to see clearly what lies ahead.

Life, in short, is complicated.

I cleared my messages and put my phone back in my pocket. I had just biked home from my shift in the emergency room, but the fog of anxiety that permeated the hospital in the spring of 2020 had followed me. To regain a sense of ease, I would first have to carefully decontaminate myself and my belongings. Whether on the front of my mask, the sides of my shoes, or on the strands of my unkempt hair, I had no doubt that I had brought the virus home with me.

I had already developed my routine, but had not yet become so habituated to it that I could perform it mindlessly. Like a student driver, I had to remain conscious of the manner and sequence of my motions. During the Ebola crisis, it was this step—the *removal* of our protective gear—that was the most important.[4] It was here that healthcare workers were most likely to become infected with the Ebola virus. If used properly, the equipment worked: it was human error that was most often our downfall. Mindless scratches of the nose and careless removals of facemasks had set off morbid cascades from which some never recovered.

This fact struck me as a strange irony. After working a long day in an intense, high-stakes environment, it might have been when we exhaled and relaxed that we were most at risk. The lifesaving intubations, the adrenaline-pumping atmosphere of a crashing patient, the anxious moments when we held our breath as we made sure our patients could breathe—these were the points at which things certainly felt most dire. Yet it was possible that it was only when everything died down—when the danger was neither palpable nor visible—that we were actually most vulnerable. The mundane act of removing one's mask was imbued with the potential of a slow-motion suicide. It would be the equivalent of successfully flying a treacherous combat mission behind enemy lines in a thunderstorm, only to crash the plane upon landing it back home on a calm and sunny day. An anticlimactic end, but one that was just as real and permanent as any other.

Still, there were limits to what we could learn from our experience with Ebola. Our current environment was very unlike our environment then. The Manhattan hospital I worked in during the Ebola crisis was designated as New York City's Ebola receiving center—we saw numerous patients thought to have the virus, and one who actually did. Wearing our normal attire through most of the day, we would pause to don our personal protective equipment only as we prepared to see a patient suspected of having the disease. Afterward, we would be received by a "doffing coach," whose entire role consisted of guiding us through the meticulous removal of our protective gear. This step of carefully removing our soiled equipment was so critical that experts did not trust us physicians to do it correctly on our own. During the Covid crisis, there was no institution designated a coronavirus receiving hospital, as every hospital had already become one by default. There was no role for a doffing coach since our workday never contained a moment free enough from the threat of Covid to actually remove our protective equipment.

And so, I never did. Long after my shift had ended, I found myself riding my bicycle through the streets of Manhattan with my hospital facemask still fixed securely to my face, its metal clips continuing to dig into the bridge of my nose until I would arrive home to finally remove it.

I entered my building and climbed the stairs to my apartment, carrying my bicycle on my shoulder. While I would normally ride the elevator, I recently began to avoid it upon returning from shift. My building included plenty of elderly tenants—neighbors whose smiles I knew well but whose names I could not produce despite years of sharing the same hallways. Through time and habituation alone, I had developed a special affection for the silver-haired lady with the wobbly blue walker, the mumbling man whose wardrobe consisted exclusively of camo and cutoff denim, and the wrinkly lady whose small talk consisted of "beautiful day, huh?" no matter the weather. Despite our exchanging little more than nods and pleasantries, these individuals had become deeply woven into the fabric of my life. It was with concern for them that I began my new routine.

My father chuckled when he learned that I was carrying my bicycle up four flights of stairs. "It's about time the donkey enjoyed some payback from his jockey," he said laughing. I rolled my eyes but secretly admired his perennially carefree and upbeat attitude.

He was raised with no electricity or running water and had witnessed several of his siblings die from the usual maladies of growing up poor in a developing country. I had always wondered whether my father had developed his cheerful outlook toward life despite the hardships he experienced, or, perhaps, precisely because of them.

As the pandemic began to roar, the death count in the emergency room climbed, and friends and family started to fall ill, I realized that I would finally put this theory to the test. Would the current tragedy make me more like my father, or less?

I pulled out the keys to my apartment. I unlocked the dead bolt first, then proceeded to release the main lock. I left my key in place and turned it to release the latch, sparing my doorknob an unnecessary touch. Returning from ten hours of wading through a cloud of Covid, I feared seeding the surfaces of my home with viral particles for my wife to pick up, as well as the potential of picking up viral particles that my wife—an OB/GYN physician actively caring for Covid patients herself—might have seeded for me.

This was, of course, during the early days of the pandemic in New York City, when the city's morgues had exceeded their capacities and bodies were being kept in refrigerated trailers parked in the street. This was when doctors and nurses were separated from their families, sending loved ones to stay at hotels or with in-laws to protect them from the virus as they shuttled to the hospital and back home. This was when medical schools graduated students before they had completed their studies in order that our front lines could be fortified with eager, if inexperienced, recruits.

This was when we were learning tremendous amounts of information about the novel coronavirus seemingly by the minute. So while future research would demonstrate that viral transmission from contaminated surfaces was rare, early studies suggested that objects like doorknobs served as important vectors of disease.[5]

Despite all this, I sometimes found the extent of my precautions excessive. "Relax, nothing's going to happen if you just turn the doorknob," I would tell myself, tired after a long day of work and eager just to get through the door. And yet, each time I learned about another dead or critically ill colleague at work, I redoubled my commitment to my routine.

The tally at just one of the two hospitals I had worked at included two physicians dead. An additional two physician assistants were admitted to the intensive care unit—one with a breathing tube down his throat so that a machine could take over his own failed attempts to breathe, another with a balloon pump in his aorta helping to make sure his exhausted heart did not give up entirely.

QS: Horrible news man. Danny is intubated right now. He came in overnight, I was taking care of him, I put him on high flow nasal cannula[6] and he was doing ok. Just woke up and checked his chart and he's fucking intubated

FN: Calling you now

Over the course of those weeks, countless doctors, physician assistants, nurses, clerks, technicians, and custodial staff had fallen ill. My phone was constantly alerting me to colleagues throughout the city falling ill with the disease. A doctor I worked alongside checked herself into the hospital one day; an overnight clerk I had just worked a shift alongside fell dead the next.

> **ES:** [sent an image referencing the death of a colleague]
> **WS:** Nooo!!
> **SE:** I really liked ▮▮▮▮▮▮, feels pretty shitty seeing that
> **WS:** I remember he smiled a lot. And was always nice
> **CA:** He was super nice and always had a positive attitude
> So awful
> **JJ:** He always had on a hoodie and a gold necklace
> **ES:** Yea and lots of rings
> **KB:** He had the most tricked out bikes

Some of these were close friends. Others were acquaintances with whom my interactions were limited to brief conversations about puncture-proof bicycle tires or up-and-coming rappers while we waited in line for coffee. Still, like the elderly residents in my apartment building, they had all, over time, become stitched into the fabric of my life.

> **ES:** Sarah was around when we were training
> She's night charge RN now
> I just was with her last Tue she was fine . . . [She's]
> now intubated in the medical ICU with Covid. Terrible.
> She's like 39 weeks pregnant
> **WS:** Omg that is horrible
> **LA:** Terrible
> Did they do a C-Section?

ES: They didn't at first—but I guess she was getting harder to ventilate (not oxygenate) and her pH was falling bc of retention, so they sectioned her just a couple hours ago.[7]

Baby intubated in neonatal ICU

AT: Shit. That's awful.

JJ: Heartbreaking

Just as one fails to notice the threads that hold a sweater together until they become loose and dangle, I began to truly appreciate the full impact of these everyday relationships only upon feeling their absence.

DD: Did you hear? ▮▮▮▮▮▮ just died.

FN: Oh shit. Seriously? That's crazy, this is too much

You sure though? ▮▮▮▮▮▮ died last week, I knew

▮▮▮▮▮▮ has been super sick but you sure you not

mixing them up?

DD: 100% sure. They both died.

For weeks to come, I would be reminded of these dead friends and colleagues as I sipped my morning coffee. In articles praising frontline workers and in tributes honoring those we lost, their faces would dot our newspapers. With so many dead, the obituaries were often presented as multi-page spreads complete with head shots and brief biographies. Somehow, they reminded me of some sort of morbid high school yearbook. Their faces smiling, we would be informed about their lives—what their personalities were like, which organizations they belonged to, and what hobbies they enjoyed. While I already knew him as an affable man with a gentle smile who was always willing to lend a hand, it was somehow strange to learn from a national publication that a surgeon I had worked alongside for years had spent time in a Buddhist monastery, was an avid rock climber, and had a degree in music.

I found myself bookmarking these articles and websites as I would come across them. It felt important that I remember the true nature of that time.

I entered my apartment and pressed some hand sanitizer into my palms. I carefully took off the disposable n95 respirator that, by then, had begun to feel like a permanent fixture of my face. I reached back to the farthest point of my head and pinched the lower elastic band, looping it over to the front of my face. Returning for the upper band, I repeated this step once more. Then, holding the mask only by its upper elastic band, I removed it, but did not toss it in the trash.

As was widely reported in the media, PPE was in short supply at the time. Our hospitals had already begun informing us that disposable equipment designed to be used for the length of a single patient interaction now had to be saved and used for days on end. Facemasks that were once freely available were now guarded by administrators equipped with lock and key. When these masks were distributed, they were often not new items, but previously used as the product of a facemask "recycling" program our hospitals had recently instituted. My wife and I feared that our institutions would soon run out of protective equipment entirely. And so, like most healthcare workers in New York City, we created a system to conserve ours.

We settled on our system not by following federal guidelines or recommendations published in peer-reviewed journals, but by sorting through text messages and browsing social media. With our normal channels of information often weeks behind the reality now thrust upon us, the vast majority of what we learned had to come from personal experience or from an informal network of friends and colleagues with direct experience with the virus themselves. A long-dormant group messaging thread of fourteen emergency physician friends from across the country had become unusually active over the past several weeks.

What we had used as a group chat to exchange news of life milestones—the birth of a child or a professional award, for example—now sprang to life as a lifeline for real-time information about the virus. We shared news articles and primary data, personal experiences with the virus that served as learning points, and asked one another to check in on family members admitted to each other's hospitals.

Pooling our experiences, we collectively saw patterns that none of us would have been able to make out on our own— when precisely to intubate a patient gasping for air, which ventilator settings we should use to optimize their chance of survival, and who, exactly, was most at risk to take a turn for the worse. We watched as the things we noted as curious personal observations later became settled knowledge about the disease.

We understood that our black and brown patients were being hit disproportionately hard by the pandemic weeks before the data confirmed it. We developed ad hoc treatment plans for disease combinations that never existed—the appropriate use of steroids and nebulizer treatments in patients who were simultaneously suffering from Covid-19 and chronic obstructive pulmonary disease, for example—before seeing our ad hoc solutions later become published as official recommendations.

With eyes and ears across nearly every hospital system in New York City, we ignored the "DO NOT DISTRIBUTE" watermarks on our hospitals' documents and shared whatever bits of information we could get our hands on. Our employment contracts contained legal clauses that treated medical knowledge as trade secrets, but we understood that keeping one another informed had the potential to save lives. And so, in some sort of underground collaborative curriculum, we used our smartphones to bypass the inefficiencies of our healthcare system.

With emergency room doctors in Seattle, Los Angeles, Houston, Denver, and almost every borough in New York engaged in a constant dialogue, we were at the bleeding edge of the pandemic. We were our own best resource and we knew it.

LA: @KB, has your ventilator rationing committee made any recs?
Are they only for placing people on ventilators? Will they make recs to take people off? Also who's on it (bioethics, pulmonary?)

KB: Not yet. But the plan is to constantly reevaluate vented

    patients w/ a plan for extubations if people start to
    decompensate

LA: So no exclusions preventing vent?
    I'm asking bc I'm gonna pass it along [at my hospital].
    Seems like next week we'll be in the same boat

DE: Sent you guys an article published in the Lancet.
    This study compared features of survivors vs non
    survivors
    It was small only 191 patients from January in Wuhan
    Only 32 were vented, of whom 31 died
    Might be useful for prognosis and selecting the sickest
    patients who have a certain number of characteristics
    that are favorable

LA: Yeah wish it had more power[8] but it looks good, going
    through the tables

KB: We have exclusions for [placing patients on]
    ventilators too
    I'll send what we have tomorrow.

It was to this informal expert network that my wife and I looked in order to determine the best strategy to conserve our protective equipment. We asked around to discover what others were doing to deal with the shortages. One colleague reported that a cousin in Singapore had mailed him a batch of n95 respirators he had lying around. Another had a shipment of masks delivered from friends in China. Colleagues in Denver, Seattle, and Houston had purchased reusable industrial respirators so that they could protect themselves in the event that their hospital's supply ran out.

Three other friends considered the merits of extending their supply of disposable masks by baking them in their ovens after their shifts to kill the contaminating virus. The idea was to use enough heat to sterilize the masks, but not so much heat that the masks would lose their integrity. They carefully discussed the precise temperature to set their ovens to and for how long they would bake their masks.

WS: I am very very worried about PPE
We have patients in open bays and don't have the equipment
I literally feel like a firefighter they are sending into a burning building or a soldier to a war zone without equipment.

AT: We are out of face masks in our trauma bays. This is absurd.

SE: I purchased my own reusable goggles and face shields.

CA: It's a real issue when your own hospital can't keep you safe.

QS: My cousin just shipped me 80 n95 masks. So if you are in the area and need some can get from me

SE: Btw, for those trying to get supplies, I was able to get my hands on this p100 with replaceable cartridges. Think this will be my last line when all n95 run out

DE: I have [one of those] with me for when we run out of supplies, but you can't even find those masks now.

BX: Per @emswami heating your N95 mask to 160F for 30 minutes will kill COVID 19 while still preserving

N95 function. Keep it off [the] metal surfaces [of your oven] with clothes pins!

Thoughts?

DE: I think it's been studied and it's legit

SE: They used e coli as the pathogen [in that study].
Would assume similar viral denaturing at those temps but COVID virus still hasn't been formally tested yet, so dunno if you can 100% extrapolate
Prob better than nothing

BX: And probs better than the brown bag I was given [at work]

Uncomfortable with the idea of cooking the masks that would protect our lives, I settled on a different approach. Preliminary studies estimated that the novel coronavirus could only survive on surfaces for up to seventy-two hours.[9] My idea, then, was to be patient. I thought we could simply put our used respirators aside for a few days and allow the virus to live its full life and die a natural death. If it took three days to effectively sterilize a mask, then four of them used in a cyclical rotation could effectively provide us with an endless supply. I proposed my idea and my colleagues agreed that the plan had merit. Individually, these were some of the best-trained doctors working in the field of emergency medicine today. If they agreed that the logic was sound, then, very likely, it was.

And so, with the blessing of a text message, my wife and I implemented our strategy. Instead of disposing of our disposable masks in the trash, we hung them on hooks nailed to our wall by the entrance of our apartment.

SE: Hope you guys are also considering your significant others at home. I've set up a dirty room/anteroom at my place to shower and store all my stuff

BX: How'd you do this (or is it a space you made formally into a bathroom/dirty room type thing?)

SE: Using an extra bathroom with big containers for all my medical supplies and scrubs. Placing shoes in "dirty" bins outside my apt, then walking in using sterile procedure and going directly to the bathroom/dirty room without touching anything (just walking in socks).
I allocated certain bags, supplies, credit cards, etc as "dirty" as well, so they aren't used outside the hospital. Basically keep outside "out" and inside "in"
Only things that cross the line are my car keys and phone, which I wipe down after every shift upon walking into my house

LA: We will all contract it if we haven't already. Gotta stay rested and as healthy as possible to keep the immune system up, minimize viral load exposures with protective gear and try to minimize/remove all contact with elderly outside the hospital
It's gonna get crazy, stay safe and good luck.

I pulled out a marker. "Last used April 13th," I wrote on a sticky note in a sort of reverse expiration date. I placed it beside today's dangling mask. Rubbing my hands with sanitizer, I then searched my wall for a used mask that was at least three days old. Finding it, I lifted it from its hook, placed it in a brown paper bag, and zippered it into my work backpack in anticipation of my next shift. I wiped down the marker with an alcohol pad and capped it once more.

As we did all this to ensure we would not run out of the equipment needed to keep ourselves and our families safe, the official position of the hospitals for which we worked was that we were engaging in hysteria; that our actions were unnecessary. In media statements and advertising campaigns, they repeatedly declared that every employee at their institution had access to any piece of PPE that was required.

When pictures of nurses at one New York City hospital wearing plastic garbage bags instead of protective medical gowns were published on the front page of our newspapers,[10] for example, a spokesperson for that hospital asked us to overlook the matter: The photograph in question "specifically shows the nurses in proper PPE underneath [the] garbage bags,"[11] we were told. A different New York City hospital, as another example, responded to criticism that they were not providing their employees with the appropriate level of PPE by dismissing the allegations as "FAKE NEWS." They claimed that they were, in fact, adhering "to the CDC guidelines at all times."[12]

While this last part was technically true, it was substantially meaningless. Despite acknowledging that "their capability to protect [medical workers] is unknown," the Centers for Disease Control and Prevention had officially sanctioned handkerchiefs, bandanas, and scarves as protective gear that healthcare providers could use as a "last resort."[13] With the country facing a critical shortage of protective equipment, it was a recommendation born not from the confidence of testing and research, but from the desperation of a limited supply. Nevertheless, as "CDC guidelines" now included practically anything to be acceptable medical gear, our hospitals did not need to provide much at all in order to truthfully claim compliance with them. It was the equivalent of the Occupational Safety and Health Administration redefining a baseball cap as an acceptable alternative to a hard hat before hearing construction foremen across the country go on to claim that their workers consistently had access to OSHA-approved protective headgear while working on-site. When the safety guidelines are devoid of substance, claims of diligent compliance with them provide little reassurance.

The reality on that ground was that our hospitals were facing severe equipment shortages and had already begun deploying questionable strategies to deal with them. These strategies had technical-sounding names like an "n95 respirator extended use plan," or a novel "ultraviolet recycling program," but we understood that these were fanciful phrases used to make us feel more confident than the situation deserved. All of us physicians in our mid to late thirties, we were raised in an era in which our institutions had pirated the English language—where the words they put forth had become untethered from any actual meaning.

We had paid for college with student loans serviced by banks that claimed to "deliver innovative financial solutions," only to see those very innovations go on to contribute to the greatest economic crisis since the Great Depression. We listened to our medical schools boast of their "deep commitment to diversity and inclusion," only to find those very same institutions systematically deny opportunities to students from diverse and disadvantaged backgrounds.[14] We had selected our residency training programs based on mission statements that proudly highlighted commitments to help "underserved and resource-poor populations," only to watch those same institutions bend over backward catering to financial donors while patients who could not afford their cancer care were sent to bankruptcy court and home foreclosure.

We were a generation that had internalized the lesson of our times. And so, despite our hospitals confidently reassuring us of their "n95 respirator extended use plans" and their "ultraviolet recycling programs," we suspected that these were words without serious meaning. We knew that, like the rest of us, our leaders too were in over their heads and did not quite know what to do. It took little more than common sense to scrutinize that single-use disposable supplies critical for personal protection ought not to be recycled or subject to extended use.

CA: They're telling us not to wear masks in the hallways because 'we're scaring the patients'

SE: Are you guys wearing n95s for evaluating each rule out case? We're being told to use just surgical masks unless doing an aerosolizing procedure

DE: There is very clearly no real plan . . .

Just like ourselves, our hospitals were scrambling. Policies changed by the hour. Early on in the crisis, for example, many hospitals had warned their employees *against* the use of facemasks while at work. Driven by a desire to be perceived as a safe place free from Covid-19, and having decided that the sight of employees wearing masks would somehow frighten patients rather than reassure them,[15] some hospitals decided to prohibit their use.[16, 17] Physicians and nurses were labeled as "insubordinate"[18]—and sometimes fired from their positions—for the act of wearing a facemask in a hospital.[19] Of course, policies that banned the use of masks inside hospitals one day turned into policies that mandated their use the next.

Protocols that guided Covid testing were similarly subject to this type of policy-whiplash. Early testing guidelines had largely restricted testing to patients who were exposed to someone who had tested positive for the virus.[20] Of course, precisely because testing was so limited at the time, the vast majority of people who had fallen ill could not claim to have been in contact with someone who had actually tested positive. And so, patients were denied testing on the grounds that the person they contracted the virus from had been unable to get tested themselves—we had, in effect, created a circular burden of proof. Soon enough, however, protocols changed such that *all* patients—regardless of the reason they had arrived to the emergency room to begin with—had to undergo Covid-19 testing before being admitted to the hospital. In this way, policies that firmly restricted testing on patients who were clearly ill with Covid one day turned into policies that firmly required testing on patients who had nothing more than hip fractures the next. Each new plan, regardless of how resolutely it flew in the face of an earlier one, was trumpeted with the same immutable confidence and assurances of safety.

KB: We are out of fentanyl[21]

WS: I heard ███████ hospital ran out of propofol[22] last week.

That true ES?

ES: Yes

We did

KB: We are running out of pumps for IV drips[23]

ES: Pumps are a problem for us too

IV Azithro[24] is running short

BX: Our whole dept is on portable vents[25] now too

RO: Apparently my hospital is basically out of tests. Isn't that kind of crazy? There are still drive through testing centers in the city. It's the weirdest experience to try and explain to patients that there aren't any tests.

SE: Same here at ███████, RO. Mostly out of tests and hospital at capacity now.

AT: ███████ is definitely picking up. It makes me so angry the lack of state and federal planning. Why are clowns representing us

WS: The testing situation is bananas

RO: I haven't been scared of the virus as a pathogen. I've been scared because it seems like no hospital administrator knows what's going on.

Rather than address our supply shortages by taking actions that would bolster our store of supplies, our country largely responded by relaxing guidelines on when these critical supplies were required to be used. Instead of invoking the Defense Production Act to manufacture more lifesaving n95 masks early in the crisis, for example, our federal agencies informed us instead that these masks were no longer necessary to be used in most circumstances.[26]

Evidence existed as early as February 2020 that Covid-19 was spread by airborne transmission—the type of transmission that an n95 mask can protect against, but that a simple surgical mask cannot.[27] Countries like Japan designed their safety protocols around such evidence and, early in the pandemic, the United States partially did as well. Initial CDC guidelines, in fact, recommended the use of n95 masks under all circumstances when treating patients who were ill with Covid-19. As supplies shriveled, however, these recommendations changed. On March 10, 2020, the CDC updated its guidelines, stating that because "the supply chain of [n95] respirators cannot meet demand," the use of simple surgical masks would be "an acceptable alternative" for healthcare workers treating Covid-19 patients.[28] It would be the equivalent of our country facing a deadly famine only to have our government respond not by supporting farmers to produce more food, but by informing citizens that due to the shortage of food, they were no longer required to eat as many meals.

RO: Just got this email from my hospital. The language is so clearly covering their ass. My boss shared some data about how droplet precautions [as opposed to airborne safety precautions] are the way to go. They are fucking us.

CA: They're saying the same at ████████

KB: Yep here too.

RO: I really think my hospital is quoting CDC guidelines about droplets because they don't want to be liable if anyone gets sick or dies and sues because they didn't have any protective gear.

ES: It's insane!! The rollback for airborne [precautions] happened right as the pandemic picked up and n95 supply dwindled
We [can't] just decide this is not airborne
In fact we now know [that it is] even more so . . .

More than a year after Covid-19 had been declared a pandemic, the CDC updated its guidelines once more. On May 7, 2021, it declared that airborne transmission of the novel coronavirus is, after all, "a key way [that] the virus is transmitted."[29]

By the end of the first twelve months of the coronavirus pandemic, more than 3,600 American healthcare workers would die of Covid-19. An investigation by Kaiser Health News and the *Guardian* would find that many of these deaths were preventable. The investigation concluded that "widespread shortages of masks and other personal protective gear, a lack of covid testing, weak contact tracing, inconsistent mask guidance by politicians, missteps by employers and lax enforcement of workplace safety rules by government regulators all contributed to the increased risk faced by healthcare workers."[30]

•   •   •

As our system convulsed, I recalled a German patient I had once cared for. On vacation in New York City, he suffered a laceration to his calf after tripping on the sidewalk. He arrived at my emergency room and was patient, pleasant, and personable. I evaluated his calf, anesthetized the area, washed his wound free of any debris and bacteria that could precipitate an infection, and stitched his wound with several sutures.

As he prepared to depart I decided, on a whim, to ask for his thoughts on his experience with the American healthcare system. He smiled, remained pleasant, and told me without a beat that the encounter was the "most disorganized, most frustrating" medical experience he had ever suffered through.

Having heard horror stories of the expense of obtaining healthcare in the United States, he told me that after he had tripped and fallen, bleeding on the sidewalk from the open gash in his leg, he was too terrified to actually go to an emergency room to seek medical care. Instead, he had returned to his hotel room to see if he could control the bleeding on his own. When he found that he could not, he tried calling various local hospitals to inquire about the cost that care in the emergency room would entail. After hours of such phone calls, bleeding through his towel as he spent much of his time on hold, it was recommended that he go to a public city hospital, where the expenses might be lower. He told me that he did this, but while waiting to be triaged, he noted a bloody needle on the floor and a generally "dirty, dangerous, crazy" atmosphere. "It certainly did not seem like anything I would expect in a first world country," he said. Determining the experience to be unsuitable, he left that hospital and walked over, still bleeding, to try his luck at the one where I happened to be working that day. Upon his arrival to my hospital, he then proceeded to wait several hours before myself or any other physician could catch up with the backlog of patients we had on that day and finally attend to his needs.

"This is America. I have traveled around the world and can say that the hospitals I have seen in poor, developing countries were better organized than what I went through today," he told me. He asked me why we, as Americans, would put up with such a system. I offered no answer. He thanked me, smiled a genuine smile, and walked out the door. I smiled back stupidly.

Considering his criticism, I had initially dismissed its harshness as the hyperbole of a man who was injured, in pain, and full of frustration as he was forced to navigate a wholly unfamiliar system. "Our system may be flawed," I thought to myself, "but at the end of the day I can't imagine that what we have is actually worse than what's being offered in developing countries. It can't be *that* bad." It wasn't until the throes of the Covid pandemic, however, that I allowed myself to entertain the notion that perhaps it was.

In that moment, I saw our experiences for what they were. We were American physicians using unstudied and unsanctioned techniques to sanitize and store single-use disposable respirators for prolonged and repeated operation. In the wealthiest country the world has ever seen, we were obtaining our supplies of lifesaving protective equipment not from our hospitals, our government, or any formal channels of operation, but from friends and relatives who mailed them to us from Singapore and China—nations we might have only recently labeled as resource-poor. We witnessed countries like Korea and Vietnam use evidence-based measures to contain the spread of the virus while our government chose to ignore that same evidence, making recommendations based on what happened to be available rather than making available what happened to be required.[31, 32, 33] We saw leaders in countries like New Zealand work to obtain protective equipment for their healthcare workers, while our president accused us of stealing ours.[34, 35]

And so, it was not until years after I had met him that I finally came to appreciate the fullness of what my German patient had offered so casually. Long before Dr. Anthony Fauci would say that America's performance during the Covid-19 crisis was "worse than most any other country"[36] on the planet, my German patient had warned me of our lagging performance. His perspective was not unduly harsh due to his unfamiliarity with our system, I came to appreciate, but it was my perspective on our system that may have been overly forgiving as a result of my own familiarity with it. The truth of that moment was that we were failing not only the standards set, say, in Germany, but that we were failing the standards set all over the world.

WS: In China and Pakistan they are wearing fully sealed
protective suits
In the goddamn USA we are asked to find a bandana in our
closet?
It's insane

PROLOGUE

DE: They did try to pull the same shit with Ebola at first. CDC said that all we needed was plastic gown and face shield mask Then those 2 ICU nurses in Texas got Ebola and the recommendations changed[37]

I finally emptied my pockets and placed my keys and wallet in a bin by the door. I wiped each surface of my phone with an alcohol pad as I prepared to cross over from the room that contained my used mask and scrubs to the room that contained the rest of my life.

Still standing by my apartment's entrance, I continued to toss my scrubs, socks, and underwear into a laundry bag. My wife asked me how my day was. I demurred with some generic non-answer—"it was okay," perhaps—and changed the subject.

Having shed my clothing, I finally dashed, completely naked, to the bathroom to shower. My wife cheered my nude dash and we both laughed. I hoped we were laughing only at the absurdity of my new routine, but it was impossible to say for sure.

As I dried off—finally free of the virus that altered the entire flow of our lives—I picked up my phone to begin what had become our new evening routine. In addition to friends and colleagues, we had family members who were affected by the virus. We called the hospitals where they were being treated to check on these patients not under my direct care.

We had started making nightly calls when we learned that my wife's father, Diego, had fallen ill. We were told that Diego had stopped breathing, that an ambulance had arrived and paramedics placed a breathing tube down his throat, and that he was transported to the nearest emergency room. Not knowing any other details about what was going on, we called the hospital to which he was transported.

The emergency room clerk picked up the phone. I remember knowing from the sound of her voice alone that Diego had died. Hearing us state his name to inform her that we were calling on his behalf, she had immediately slowed her voice and relaxed her cadence. It was the familiar calmness that those of us who work in the emergency room allow ourselves only in the face of death. In a place designed to prioritize urgent matters among a vast pool of urgent matters, there is only a single matter over which nothing can be prioritized.

Research has shown that, on average, an emergency physician is interrupted more than a dozen times per hour.[38] We may be handed a concerning EKG while speaking with a patient about their broken ankle. We may be asked to step away from a patient suffering from pneumonia upon receiving notification that an ambulance is about to bring us a person who was struck by a car. We may be in the middle of a conversation with a patient who has been having thoughts of suicide only to be asked to step out of the room to quickly attend to a patient who began suffering a seizure.

When a patient has died, however, we are generally left undisturbed. Our colleagues will cover our work and respond to our emergencies in order to permit us to attend to the delicate task of speaking with the family of the deceased. They will absorb our distractions in order that we can provide the focus and attention that such a moment deserves; it is only when someone has died, then, that we allow ourselves a bit of calm.

And so, we permit ourselves to slow our voice and relax our cadence when speaking with the family members of our dead patients.

JJ: How is Vivian's dad doing?

FN: Thanks everyone. He didn't make it. We really appreciate everyone's thoughts and help. He was only 59. Please be careful.

KB: Farz—give my love to Viv. I'm sorry.

Hours after he was buried in a small and socially distanced ceremony, we received a call that Diego's sister, Maria, was being rushed to the emergency room. Appearing relatively well just hours earlier when she attended her brother's funeral via video chat, she had now found herself in much the same position that her brother was in the week before.

FN: Hey guys, Vivian's aunt is now intubated and at ████████ hospital in [Brooklyn]. Do we know anyone that might work there? Thanks

RO: Shit that's awful.

CA: I'm sorry Farz, thinking about you and Vivian

JJ: Omg I'm so sorry, I'll ask around

KB: Farz—I'm sorry man. I don't know anyone.

WS: Got Farzon a connect. We have deep networks within NYC people. And really anywhere. We can almost always crowd source a connection. Keep em coming if needed. I can text and email away from home!!

We called the emergency room that was caring for her. The doctor in charge was the friend of a colleague. Knowing that having personal ties to our patients makes it more challenging to care for them, I understood that we had just made his evening more difficult.

He took a deep breath and filled us in on the situation. He told us that despite her breathing at a rate three times faster than was normal, the oxygen levels in Maria's blood were only about a third of what they should have been. He informed us that like her brother before her, she too had to have a breathing tube placed. Soon breathing with the assistance of a mechanical ventilator, she was to be transferred to the intensive care unit.

Because of her critical state, our phone calls to Maria's care team became a nightly occurrence. The only physicians in our respective families, my wife and I served primarily as medical liaisons. Fluent in the jargon that healthcare providers seem to find impossible to avoid, we would receive updates from the care team and then translate and relay those updates to the rest of my wife's family.

Maria required the constant infusion of two medications maxed out to their highest levels to keep her blood pressure from plummeting, as well as a mechanical ventilator to breathe for her. The first few days of her hospital stay were eventful and required plenty of explaining. Our role was critical to Maria's husband, son, and daughter understanding what was occurring.

Within a few days, however, Maria's illness was severe but stabilized. While she remained moments away from death, days would go by with neither improvement nor decline. And so, our liaison had become strikingly easy.

"Nothing's really changed since yesterday," we were told by the care team this evening. "Nothing's really changed since yesterday," we would then tell Maria's husband and children.

Understanding the grim prognosis, we walked a careful line between expressing our hopes of what was to come and our realistic understanding of what was likely to. Over the years, I have learned the hard way that offerings of hope must be carefully titrated and calibrated. Too little hope, of course, and one can prematurely crush another's world. Too much hope, however, and one can create a false optimism that can only lead to a more devastating experience later.

"We have to hope for the best, but she's super sick now and that is certainly a possible outcome," we told Maria's children when they asked my wife and me if we thought their mother was going to die.

As we hung up the phone, we heard a coughing fit from the other side of our apartment wall. Over the past several days, it was clear that one of our neighbors had fallen ill. My wife and I had tried to pinpoint the source of the sound. The origin of the cough seemed to change throughout the course of the day. At some points, it sounded as if it were coming from the other side of our bedroom wall, from the young woman with the Russell terrier. At other times, however, the cough sounded as if it were coming from above, from the neighbor whose apartment sat directly atop ours. At still other times, it seemed to surround us, as if the booming cough were coming from everywhere all at once. Somehow it was fitting.

Converging on us from seemingly every angle, the sound of Covid had come to embody our experience with the disease itself.

I took one final glance at my phone before putting it away.

QS: Anybody have any good news regarding any of the patients they have admitted w/ Covid so far?

BX: I stopped following up to be honest

KB: None

QS: Ya same. I have one guy who is 30 who was never intubated. But he ended up doing well enough to be discharged with home oxygen

DE: Wasn't my patient but a hospital I work at just discharged a 92 year old

ES: We've discharged some but most of them just live on the ventilator for a long time it seems.

ES: Then die

KB: Yep

JJ: Yikes that is terrifying

ES: It's a mess here

KB: This is a wild time. I'm very happy to have you guys.

RO: Me too. Love you guys.

WS: Guys. Is it bad to use work health insurance for a psychiatrist or therapist?
I'm gonna need actual help to deal with this. That is pretty clear to me already

After having more than my fill of the virus for the day, I powered my phone off.

•   •   •

I began to prepare dinner. As I did, Vivian came over to show me a video op-ed by Nicholas Kristof published in the *New York Times*. It was an inside look into a busy emergency room in New York City during the pandemic.

There were shaky camera angles and professional editorial cuts. The video was set to emotional music and was somberly narrated. We were shown critically ill patients crowded into hallways while doctors and nurses spoke in tense and urgent voices. The inescapable cacophony of beeping machines, overhead announcements, ringing phones, and human distress caused a physical response in my stomach. I watched in awe. I was stunned. "God, that looks insane," I remarked to my wife.

Only later did I realize that the video was simply a narrated version of my own lived experience. I had come home from a busy shift in a New York City emergency room only hours ago.

It can be difficult to see the composite of our life instead of how we experience it day to day. The routine serves as camouflage—we often do not inspect and analyze things that we are intimately familiar with. Sometimes we need to see familiar things from a new angle to appreciate them for what they really are.

I recall once, while I was learning Spanish, coming across the word "sombre," which is Spanish for "shade." I immediately appreciated that it was the basis for "sombrero"—that a hat was nothing more than a shade maker we place on our heads. The insight served no functional purpose. Nevertheless, it was enriching—it was the type of connection that helped me appreciate the depth and nuance of the language I was beginning to pick up. It was also the type of connection made possible precisely because of my lack of familiarity. It would be difficult for a native speaker to pause, dissect and inspect each word, and connect the dots in the way that I was forced to do. And so, where insiders can claim expertise, I learned, outsiders benefit from a fresh analysis.

In this way, as I was watching this video about my own experience from a neutral, outsider's perspective, something clicked. Over the years, I had gotten used to my job. I had gotten acclimated to the sights and sounds of human lives in disarray and the turbulent efforts to address them. Now, in an instant, I was able to see it for what it really was.

"That's insane," I had remarked about what was ostensibly my own day-to-day experience.

What stayed with me long after the video ended, however, was not that it felt so familiar to my experience in the emergency room during the pandemic, but that it felt so familiar to my experience in the emergency room in general. Except for the ubiquitous PPE unique to the pandemic, the video somehow felt as if it could have been a scene from any emergency room at any time. The video was not a wake-up call to my past several weeks, then, but to my past several years.

Filmed in a hospital I had never stepped foot in, it was both instantly recognizable and deeply familiar. Watching it felt like having an out-of-body experience or peering into an alternate reality where things were somehow different, yet exactly the same. The nurses wore a different brand of scrubs and the walls were painted a different color, but the rapidly beeping monitors still announced that a patient was teetering at the edge of her body's limits, the stretchers stacked in hallways still indicated there existed more patients than resources, and the strained voices with which the doctors and nurses spoke still signified that the staff was working a few steps beyond their point of exhaustion. It was all so familiar that I did not feel as if I was watching the video so much as experiencing it.

Slowly and over time, I had gotten acclimated to it all. Somehow, writhing bodies and pained groans had become normalized and lost their punch. The video hit me in the gut.

And so, while it was intended to show us the intense and extreme lengths healthcare professionals went to as we battled the coronavirus, my takeaway instead was to finally appreciate just how intense and complicated our daily experience has *always* been.

This is not to diminish the Covid-19 pandemic. Without any doubt, the pandemic was bigger than anything we had previously encountered. After all, we were confronted with a virus that spread through the air and killed many of those it infected. We knew little about the disease, and less about how to treat it. Scores of patients died. Friends and colleagues did, too. Family members were not spared. I pronounced patients dead and I attended socially distanced funerals. More than a few emergency physician friends felt the need to seek psychiatric care for the first time in their lives. Several expressed their desire to leave the practice of medicine entirely.

Without a doubt, the pandemic left its enduring mark.

But the truth is, the pandemic did not change the nature of our work. While the pandemic may have made things more difficult, it did not necessarily make them different. The most challenging circumstances I faced during the pandemic, in fact, had little to do with the virus itself.

In the opening spring of the Covid-19 crisis, I diagnosed an elderly patient with a severe case of the virus. His oxygen levels were dipping and his blood tests indicated a poor prognosis. What made my job difficult, however, was not the medical care I would provide him. It was easy enough to place the order for the Tylenol that would address his fever and to strap on the noninvasive ventilator that would treat his respiratory distress.[39] What made my job so difficult, then, was everything that surrounded the medical care we provided.

The patient had asked me what to expect. I told him the truth: that it was impossible to predict the future, that many people in his condition would go on to do well, but that a good deal of others did not. I told him that, at the moment, he was quite ill, that his situation was grave, and that we would be admitting him to the intensive care unit. I went on to tell him that he was in good hands and that we would be doing everything we could to ensure that he would do as well as our science, technology, and humanity allowed.

What made my job difficult was reconciling the stoicism he expressed in his words with the fear that was evident in his eyes. What made my job difficult was seeing him nod his head in appreciation when I told him that he "was in good hands" and that we would "do everything we could," despite knowing that our good hands doing everything they could had little power to affect his ultimate outcome. What made my job difficult was deciding precisely how to word the truths I had conveyed. Was it enough to leave things vague and simply tell him that "many" people in his position "did well" while "a good deal of others did not"? Or, was it important to communicate specifically that I feared that he was more likely to fall into the latter camp? That what I meant when I said that "a good deal of others" did not go on to "do well" was that they would die? Where, precisely, was the line between informing and empowering him, and simply being cruel?

And so, in the midst of a once-in-a-century airborne pandemic that would go on to kill millions around the world, what actually made my job so difficult was deciding the best way to frame a conversation.

In the first summer of the Covid crisis, I announced a time of death in the company of two nurses, one respiratory therapist, one patient technician, two paramedics, and a cold, naked body. The medical part of my job was not difficult. My patient had lost his pulse more than an hour before I had ever met him—the entirety of the medical care that I provided for this patient was to simply recognize that he was dead and declare him as such.

What made the practice of medicine so difficult, then, was that it was a practice involving people.

The paramedics told me that the wife of my dead patient was on her way to the hospital. They told me that she had been driving her husband to the hospital after he had begun complaining of some difficulty breathing. They told me that they picked him

up on the side of the road, however, as he had lost consciousness while en route, before he and his wife could make it to their
destination. They told me that they had arrived at the scene only
to find this patient already dead, that they began chest compressions in the shoulder lane of the expressway as the patient's
young daughter looked on from inside her mother's car.

What made my job difficult here was watching my patient's
wife walk toward the room where I would inform her that her
husband had died, only to appreciate that in addition to carrying
her young daughter in her arms, she was visibly pregnant as well.
What made my job difficult was hearing her say "no, I am alone
here, it was just my husband and me. We've only been in this
country for a few months," when I asked her if there was anyone she could call who could come support her during that difficult time. What made my job difficult was noticing her young
daughter perk up and look at me when I uttered the words, "yes,
he has died," in response to her mother's request for confirmation of what I had just said. While the daughter was oblivious
to much of what was happening before that moment—happily
playing with her dolls while her mother shook and sobbed—it
was clear that as much as she was unfazed by everything that
came before it, those words held meaning for her.

And so, having just laid my hands on a cold gray man before declaring his death, what actually made my job so difficult
had nothing to do with medicine, but simply with wondering
how much a four-year-old might have actually understood in
that moment, and how much she might remember.

•　　•　　•

In the first autumn of the Covid crisis, I cared for a patient with an abnormal heart rhythm. His heart was beating not only irregularly, but also too fast. Left untreated, he could have suffered a heart attack, lost his blood pressure, and died. Nevertheless, it was simple enough to interpret the results of his EKG and administer the medications that would slow and stabilize his heart. In fact, my patient had told me what was going on and what I needed to do to treat it himself.

"I was diagnosed with an atrial flutter in the summer," I recall him saying. "We were scheduled to do an ablation to fix it in August but I lost my job as a pilot because of the pandemic. The whole airport pretty much shut down because nobody is flying and we all lost our jobs. When I lost my job I also lost my health insurance, though, so I was never able to get the procedure done." He told me how, unemployed, uninsured, and anxious about the costs that a visit to the hospital would entail, he avoided coming to the emergency room for hours despite his racing heart. "They told me someone from the hospital's financial counseling services would call me, but nobody ever did," he told me with tears welling in his eyes. "I can't tell you how many voicemails I left but nobody ever called me back."

What made my job difficult was being forced to simply nod and agree with him, while understanding that I was part of the very system that had created his dilemma. What made my job difficult was recognizing that I would only be able to solve one of his problems at the expense of exacerbating another—the medicines I would use to fix his heart rate would generate a bill that he could not afford. What made my job difficult was following his hospital course in my computer's electronic medical record long after I had admitted him, only to learn that three days into his hospital stay, my patient's heart rhythm changed once more, this time into an even more dangerous one. Ultimately, his heart would stop beating. Hospital staff would have to administer chest compressions along with a cocktail of several medications in order to reel him back from a brief brush with death. Of course, the entire circumstance he found himself in—including his death and subsequent resurrection—would have never been necessary had he simply been able to obtain the procedure he needed when his problem had first been identified months earlier.

What made my job so difficult, then, was knowing that there now existed a member of my community who could count "death" among his life's experiences, because of nothing other than a systems failure.

In the first winter of the Covid pandemic, I cared for an elderly husband and wife who had both arrived at my emergency department ill with symptoms of Covid-19. By this time, drugs to treat the disease had started to become available. The Food and Drug Administration had authorized the emergency use of monoclonal antibodies—intravenous medications that would bind to the virus and blunt its replication, helping to prevent further clinical deterioration from the disease. What studies were available at the time demonstrated that the therapy was effective and that it contained few side effects.[40, 41] It was, of course, not a difficult decision to offer it.

I called my hospital's pharmacy to arrange for the infusions. The pharmacist agreed that my patients both fit the criteria

that would make them eligible for the drug's use, then proceeded to ask me which of them I believed should receive it. I
thought that I had misheard. "Oh, actually, they both need it,"
I attempted to clarify. The pharmacist then informed me that
due to a nationwide shortage of the medication at the time,
our entire hospital had been receiving only handfuls of doses
delivered several times per week. At the time of my phone call,
she said, there was a single dose left in our hospital.

What made my job difficult was having to sit down with
this husband and wife and explain that one of them would
be getting the treatment, while the other would have to be
sent home without it. I had to navigate an impossible ethical dilemma with no framework to guide me. There were no
rules—of course, there *could* be no rules—that would dictate
the correct course of action here. Indeed, there was no such
thing as a "correct" course of action at all.

What actually made my job so difficult, then, was knowing that I was faced with a situation for which there existed
no correct course of action, and then having to pursue one
anyway.

In short, what made my job so difficult in each of these
scenarios was precisely the same sort of thing that had always
made it difficult.

And so, in this way, Covid-19 might have been new, but
the complex web of social, emotional, bureaucratic, and philosophical situations that we had to work through in order to treat
it was not. Long before the Covid crisis we had had to navigate
difficult conversations with our patients, we had to tell family
members that their loved ones had died, we had to witness the

impossible cruelty of our healthcare system, and we had to navigate ethical and moral dilemmas for which there existed no solutions. The pandemic did not change the nature of our work. It did not make life in the emergency room qualitatively different, but quantitatively so.

The Covid-19 pandemic was not different, then, but *more*. If the volume in the emergency room during the coronavirus pandemic cranked up to an earth-rattling thirteen out of ten, the reality was that it had always been an unsustainable eleven out of ten beforehand.

Even before the pandemic, we were stretched beyond our limits. Even before the pandemic, we knew that—at their best—the frameworks and schemas we used to make sense of the countless tragedies we witnessed were not adequate to the task. Even before the pandemic, our system was failing the people it was designed to serve. Even before the pandemic, we were losing healthcare workers to the occupational hazards of our work—not to a contagious virus, but to burnout and suicide.[42]

April 2021

JJ: Do you guys remember ▮▮▮▮▮▮▮? [He graduated residency a few years before us] and worked as an attending at ▮▮▮▮▮▮ for a little bit before he went out to California.

JJ: I just saw on Facebook that he committed suicide. It's so sad

JJ: [sent an image]

BX: Fuck

WS: Oh man. That's so sad.

January 2018

ES: [Sent a link to an article that begins: "Yesterday afternoon another young doctor jumped to her death in NYC. She landed at the entrance of the building where she lived."]

SE: Shit. Was this at ███████ [Hospital]?

BX: Yeah. Again.

BX: They had another one recently, too

KB: Thanks for sending this ES.

PK: We knew [about this] at ███████ because we had to call around and account for all our residents [to make sure they were all still alive].

FN: So crazy

PK: It's horrible!

UP: Thanks for sharing. Love to you all.

Covid-19 was not a wrecking ball, then, but a magnifying glass. It did not break American medicine but reveal it for what it has always been.

Long before the pandemic had ever hit, our experiences were challenging, strange, and discomfiting. Long before the pandemic had hit, our routine was to encounter impossible situations for which there exist no answers, and then, to answer them. Routinely, we take part in tragedies that cannot be explained, scenarios that exist beyond the sphere of logic, and circumstances that we do not have the tools to address. Our work is nothing less than a beautifully crafted jigsaw puzzle short several pieces and with an additional few thrown in that do not fit.

Too often, instead of learning to appreciate this tapestry for what it is, we simply ignore the missing and discomfiting bits, pretending they do not exist. In much the same way that I demurred when my wife asked me how my day in the emergency room went upon my returning home from work, we often avoid and deflect the things that make us uncomfortable. We are not doing ourselves any favors. There is inherent value in slowing down and seeing things for what they really are. After all, one can see a silver lining only if one faces the clouds.

And so, if the video of someone else's experience in the emergency room was eye-opening, I had to consider that perhaps my own experiences were as well. It was time to take a closer look.

With all this in mind, I initially wanted to write a story about my experience as an emergency room doctor during the Covid pandemic. My intention was to write about our circumstances in order to highlight the nuances, emotional depths, and complex beauty that is hidden but inherent in those moments.

What follows, however, is a story about a routine experience I had as an emergency physician in a pre-Covid world.

I intentionally chose to write about the pre-pandemic world for the reason I just described: it is our normal world that deserves the most reflection. A story about my experiences during the age of Covid would have been easy to dismiss as a mix of emotions, dilemmas, and paradoxes exclusive to an exceptional circumstance. This is not the case. The way we experienced the pandemic was a direct consequence of how we were living before it. And as our lives were profound and complicated before the pandemic, so too will they be after it passes. It would not serve us to pretend otherwise.

The real story of the Covid-19 pandemic was how, through its extreme nature, it forced us to shake up the normal flow of our lives. It forced us to pause, take a step back, and see our lives not for the strange and challenging episode they were during the pandemic, but for the strange and challenging reality they have always been. The story of the Covid-19 pandemic is not one to be told through a highlight reel, then, but by reflection in a rearview mirror.

So what follows is a story about a real experience that is simultaneously routine and exceptional. It is the story of a normal day in the emergency room that is, of course, anything but. It is an attempt to peer into that life and take a sober look around. Like changing perspective to newly appreciate the stars in the night sky that have always been there, I hope that describing this experience can uncover profound new perspectives that we may have previously missed. Ultimately, it is an attempt to examine life.

Lastly, a forewarning: my story contains no answers. What it does is simply present life as it is. I invite you to join me with an open mind to see the same old sights with fresh new eyes. I hope it is as enlightening for you to read as it was for me to write.

PART I

Life always bursts the boundaries of formulas.

—Antoine de Saint Exupéry, *Flight to Arras*

ONE

DEATH'S HERALD

At the tail end of an overnight shift, in a small community hospital in one of New York City's outer boroughs, our little healthcare army—about a dozen nurses, three patient technicians, one physician assistant, an indefatigable medical scribe, and myself—reeled as the red phone rang. The 1980s-era corded phone had no caller ID, but none was needed. The red phone was death's herald, and calls from it always meant that someone had died or was dying, and that person was on their way to us.

The charge nurse grabbed a notepad as she listened to the muffled voice on the other end of the line. Static made it difficult for her to hear, but she squinted her eyes and peered ahead intently as if the voice were a blurry image she could not quite see. Two decades into the twenty-first century and we somehow still lacked a reliable phone connection. I read her transcription in real time as she scribbled her notes:

43yo F. Pulseless x 30 mins. CPR in progress. Intubated. ETA 6 mins.

Each of us sighed and began preparing for our arrival. The ambulance was bringing a dead woman to our emergency room. Beyond that, the death of this particular woman was without recourse—she would remain dead.

This was no criticism of the skill of the paramedics or of ourselves, but simply commentary on the limits of the human body.

Some dead patients *can* be brought back to life. Centuries of rigorous scientific research, crossed with centuries of ingenuity, crossed with the occasional wanton good luck have endowed us with such magical tools as endotracheal intubation, central intravenous lines, and epinephrine. We can breathe for people who have stopped breathing, refill a tank of blood for those who have dipped down to "E," and even trick a defeated heart into beating once again. Through the miracle of modern medicine, a very small number of dead patients can be resurrected and go on to tell the story of that time they came back from beyond. That is, of course, the holy grail. There is no better feeling than doctor-as-resurrectionist.

This particular dead patient, however, would not give us such satisfaction. This patient, we all knew, would remain dead; that verdict was already made, and even the best that medicine had to offer could make no appeal. Our patient was without a pulse for thirty minutes and counting. After such a long duration of the heart failing to beat properly, the brain loses oxygen for too long a time for any meaningful chance of recovery. When the brain has died, the rest, of course, is a futile exercise.

Nevertheless, we donned our gloves and prepared our equipment. Perhaps there was a communication error and the patient was pulseless for three, not thirty, minutes. Maybe there was indeed a pulse, but the paramedic simply could not feel it. Maybe the patient was found at the bottom of a frozen lake, making her a rare exception to the normal rules that govern when, precisely, it is that death becomes irrevocable ("you're not dead until you're warm and dead," the teaching goes). Or maybe I was relying on science too much and a miracle would occur. After all, one thing I have learned from working in the emergency room is that nothing is as certain as it may seem.

The only certainty that remained after the red phone rang was that our ten-hour overnight shift would now extend well into the morning.

As the sound of the arriving sirens grew louder, any uncertainties that did remain began to evaporate. From the speed that the ambulance drove into the loading bay and the ambiguous sound of determined voices coming from inside the truck, it was clear no miracle had occurred. We were to receive another dead body that, with or without any chance of recovery, we had to act upon.

As the automatic doors opened and the frigid winter air rushed through our emergency department, the patient was wheeled in on a stretcher.

Each player scrambled to execute their role—plugging in wires, inserting intravenous lines, and cutting off clothes with trauma shears. Contrary to television depictions of such moments, there was no shouting. Outwardly, there was barely any palpable drama at all. Our team functioned in silence so that the paramedics could fill us in.

> **Me:** Okay, guys, talk to me, what's going on?
>
> **Paramedics:** Hey, Doc—we got a forty-three-year-old female. She was complaining of abdominal pain and chest pain to her husband during the day, then she felt short of breath so she called 911. When we got there she was totally normal, walkie-talkie—she looked fine actually. We got an 18-gauge IV in the left antecube and started giving her some fluids, but then she suddenly collapsed. She was pulseless, EKG was in asystole, so we started CPR, tubed her, and gave her five rounds of epi.[1]

Winston and Lewis were two of the best paramedics I knew. They were the good guys you hated to see, the type of guys who have waded through scenes of blood and vomit with nothing but surgical gloves and grit. The type of guys who seemed to always bring good energy and bad news. I trusted them entirely, and notions of a communication error or a missed pulse rapidly vanished.

> **Me:** How long has she been pulseless in total at this point?
>
> **Paramedics:** Almost forty minutes now.
>
> **Me:** Did you get a pulse back at any point or was she pulseless the entire time?

Paramedics: No pulse at any point.

Me: Sounds like you guys did everything—what else is there to do?

Paramedics (still out of breath, sweating from the last half hour of nonstop movement, visibly defeated): Ah, shit. The paperwork?

One of the strangest things about medicine is that things seem to have their own momentum. Often, things happen and it is not entirely clear why they do. The paramedics, myself, the nurses—we all knew this patient had no chance at survival. And yet staring at the sad, naked body on the gurney, her mouth agape, a breathing tube the size of a garden hose protruding from between her lips, our doing nothing would have felt unconscionable.

Winston and Lewis could have called a time of death en route, and they would have earned the right to do so. They tried to pump life into her dusky body and could have credibly said, "We tried, we could not get her back, so she is dead." With the patient having just arrived to the hospital, though, and us yet to lay a finger on her, we had not yet earned that right. This was purely emotional reasoning—no matter what we did, the outcome would be no different. Yet it would feel inappropriate to get started on a death certificate without having so much as touched her.

I turned back to the patient. Her plump body was stripped nude to allow us to look for injuries and treat her with various needles, pharmaceuticals, and electrical conductors. Blood and plastic tubing oozed from her arms. Her naked body was slumped to the side, half falling off the gurney in a position so twisted that even I winced in discomfort.

The indignity of medicine can be profound.

A nurse instinctively readjusted her. "C'mon, let's get you fixed up," she warmly offered to the dead body as she grabbed her shoulders, straightened out her flopping neck, and half-draped her with a hospital gown. The remark was unconscious and reflexive. The indignity of death was casually met by the empathy of the living. We would not dare stand too near this patient in an elevator for fear of invading her personal space, but now we freely poked and prodded her naked body while covering it up and whispering kind reassurances to her unhearing ears.

A common misconception of medical professionals is that our natural emotions become replaced by a cool, calculating demeanor. Where someone else might feel sadness or panic, for example, a paramedic, nurse, or emergency room doctor is thought to block out his or her feelings and take action. The truth, however, is that those powerful visceral emotions are not replaced by an indifferent calm. They are simply papered over by it. In other words, under the surface of a calm operator there still exist very raw, very real, human emotions. They always make their presence felt—invisible but boiling, like magma below the surface of a dormant volcano.

It is a phenomenon I imagine we share with all those whose jobs bring them face-to-face with death—from firefighters to police officers and even combat soldiers. Panic is self-defeating, and it can be controlled, but no amount of training overrides the body's highly evolved, instinctive reaction to death itself. We can slow our heart rates and bring a calm, algorithmic approach to our thought processes, but the pit of our stomachs will independently acknowledge death and keep a check on our humanity.

Such is the case whenever I am confronted with a dead body. A dead, naked body, of course, is an extraordinarily sad sight. Yet it is not sad in the way that death itself is sad—which is to say, sad because a human soul has extinguished. That particular sadness comes later. That particular sadness happens when speaking with the family or going through that patient's belongings. That sadness comes from learning the human details that personify that body. That sadness comes from going through a patient's wallet to search for a next of kin long after the person has died, and coming across a sandwich shop rewards card or a to-do list. That the now-dead patient was only two visits away from a free twelve-inch sub or had to buy cat food on his way home from work personifies that dead body. Index cards and Post-it notes transform. They turn sixty-two-year-old males with past medical histories of diabetes mellitus and hyperlipidemia, who suffered cardiac arrests from left anterior descending coronary artery occlusions, into men named Carl who used to enjoy roast beef sandwiches and loved their cats.

Before we get to that point, however, we are faced with nameless vessels. Devoid of any narrative or intention, an anonymous dead body is sad in a distinctly pedestrian, matter-of-fact way—a previously lithe, elegant body, reduced to limp flesh. Everything not securely fixed to the trunk—limbs, female breasts, male genitalia—flops around purposelessly with each chest compression like ribbons tied to an air conditioner at an appliance store. Hands that may have previously played the piano or legs that used to climb mountains become inert and rubbery.

In this way, an anonymous dead body ultimately evokes a deeply pathetic sadness. But they exist, and we are entrusted to do right by them. And so, while the dusky body in front of us simply lay there inert, it nevertheless demanded action.

> **Me:** Okay, thanks so much, guys. Alexandria, could you please start the stopwatch. Danny, could you use the GlideScope to confirm the ET tube is still in place?[2] Daris, can you get a second IV on the right side, biggest one you could get, please—and let's also draw off labs and check the glucose at the same time. Let's continue CPR until the next epi and pulse check.

Death is bewildering on many levels. When I was a medical student, however, it was the medical treatment of death that I found particularly curious. The moments just before death can be wildly different—thousands of different diseases, each with dozens of different treatment options. But once that threshold is crossed—once "very sick" becomes "dead"—everything converges into a single pathway. Ultimately, there is one treatment protocol for death: CPR, oxygen, and a small handful of medications. Unlikely as it seems, whether the cause was a heart attack or malaria, the treatment of death is always the same. And so, just as death is the final landing place for all the divergent and individual lives that came before it, the medical treatment of death, too, is a final common denominator.

Like a group of honeybee worker drones, our little team was buzzing in action. A flurry of activity, but organized and with each honeybee knowing exactly his or her role. Despite understanding that we were trying to pollinate a stone, we nevertheless swarmed the lifeless rock.

Me: Were you able to check the glucose in the field?[3]
Paramedics: Yup. Normal.
Me: Any past medical problems?
Paramedics: None.
Me: Any idea what might have happened?
Paramedics: No clue. She was fine and then she collapsed.
Me: Does she have any family?
Paramedics: Her husband is on his way over right now.

Ah, okay, now *this* was why we were doing all this. Finally, here lay the justification for our otherwise futile activity. The dead woman would certainly stay dead, but we would still affect a life.

TWO

MEDICAL DEGREE VS. PUPPY DOG

Like every other premedical student, I became a doctor because I wanted to help people.

Like "paradigm shift" and "ideate" in other fields, "help people" is the medical world's very own meaningless catchphrase. Its emptiness reveals the lack of clarity at its root. This lack of clarity in the very idea that propelled many of us to enter our profession leaves many doctors scrambling to find meaning in their job later in their careers.

Entering medicine with good intentions but without specifics about whom I wanted to help or how I would go about doing it, I was soon surprised at how hard it was to truly help anyone at all.

The idea of a sick person coming to see a doctor, being diagnosed and treated, and later leaving cured and satisfied is woefully quaint. Aside from some great strides made with antibiotics and preventative vaccines, for example, strikingly few of our treatments are slam dunks. Simultaneously, modern medicine is incredibly advanced and stubbornly Stone Age: we may be able to give you a literal new heart, but we have little to offer for your debilitating chronic back pain.

If this paradox is easy to understand, it is difficult to digest. It results, often, in dissatisfaction. Patients with minor complaints often come to the emergency room hoping for cures that are beyond our ability. My reassurances that sprained ankles will heal, flu symptoms will resolve, and that narcotics are no better for knee pain than over-the-counter ibuprofen, are often met with skepticism or disappointment.

The sentiment is entirely understandable. Like a nation unsettled by the realization that the same government that could land a man on the moon could not get clean water to a major American city after a hurricane, we have a hard time processing medicine's very real limitations. Patients who read about groundbreaking advances like face transplants and genetic modification have a difficult time appreciating our impotence in the face of many common ailments.

"My aunt just got two new knees like the bionic woman," one patient once told me, "but you're saying you really got nothing for this cold that's killing me?"

We really have nothing. When miracles are commonplace, "watchful waiting" can be difficult to accept.

Those with major medical problems do not fare all that much better. Even those who experience modern medicine's true miracles inevitably become exasperated upon appreciating the extent of the fine print involved. Like an omnipotent genie slowly realizing that his supreme power comes with a set of inescapable handcuffs, it takes time for patients to realize that their miraculous procedure includes a set of severe limitations.

For example, when one is faced with certain death, a lifesaving liver transplant is a no-brainer. Yet the euphoria of a second shot at life dims as it becomes clear that this second life will be far more restricted than the first. The frequent hospitalizations, doctor visits, and complete ban on alcohol dispirit many. For the remainder, the incessant needle sticks, blood draws, and chronic medications with their chronic side effects usually do the trick. Patients appreciate the treatments we are able to offer them, but, at the same time, they can become frustrated.

Understanding they've been sent to the emergency room by their primary care doctor for IV antibiotics to treat a severe infection, for example, these patients sometimes refuse the placement of that very IV upon arrival. "I *hate* needles, don't go sticking me with any!" they might say, stubbornly refusing our offers to help. Eventually, they almost always relent, sighing and extending their arm to expose their veins, deeply upset at the terms of the bargain they have agreed to. "Fine, I'll give you one shot to get the IV but if you miss that's it," they may say, negotiating the terms by which we are permitted to provide the medications that will save their lives. Regardless of how many attempts it may take, of course, they generally allow us to proceed, understanding that it is what they need to do to stay alive.

At first glance, this type of behavior may seem absurd. Many doctors and nurses, myself included, have become frustrated with these "difficult" patients. *Let me do my job so that you can be helped!* we might think. *We both know you need this—this is what you came here for to begin with—so why go through this charade? You're only making things harder for both of us.*

But these patients are not merely acting out. Neither are they acting irrationally. Those of us who become frustrated have failed to put ourselves in their shoes. To live the life of many chronically ill patients is to live a restricted life. In such a world, we too would complain about our tedious predicament. We too would be nostalgic for a life that was once much richer. But we too would ultimately relent, knowing it is what we need to stay alive.

A life of mere survival is a life of gray, muted hues. Ultimately, this life is the reality of even our best modern achievements. The truth is that we do not liberate these patients from their disease, but reduce their sentences down to life on parole. Our most incredible medical miracles prolong life at the cost of living.

While most of the patients who develop frustrations with what we have to offer do not direct their dissatisfaction toward their physicians, they are dissatisfied nonetheless. "Ah, my situation is terrible and there is nothing that can be done, but I guess I understand that science has its limits; thanks anyway, Doc," is not exactly the euphoria of healing the ill that I had in mind when I decided I wanted to "help people."

And so, it was under these circumstances that soon after graduating residency—frustrated by our collective inability to help our patients to the degree that I wished we could—I began playing a game I call "Medical Degree versus Puppy Dog."

After each patient I saw, I would ask myself: Would this patient's problem be better handled by myself, with a decade of rigorous medical training and board certification in emergency medicine, or by a yellow Labrador with a wagging tail?

I kept a written tally. That "Medical Degree" would mostly win was little reassurance. That it was a close competition at all was disturbing. Furthermore, that I would occasionally wrap up a shift and realize that "Medical Degree" had lost to "Cute Puppy" was a more profound statement of modern American medicine than anything I have ever read in any newspaper's op-ed page.

The game is effectively this: Many of our patients are already well aware of the limits of modern medicine. Many of the minorly ill already know deep in their hearts that we cannot cure them. The majority of those suffering from chronic illness, having lived with their problem for years, know their situation better than their doctors do. They appreciate our treatments, of course, but ultimately what they are really looking for is to simply feel better. These people want comfort and reassurance. They simply want to be listened to and to have their story be heard.

Dogs are excellent at this. They lie on our laps and express their affection. They are deeply concerned with what we are feeling. They allow us to tell our stories and are never in a rush to leave our side. So while they provide no breakthroughs and certainly administer no pharmaceuticals, they nevertheless provide a terrific comfort. Solving nothing, they still provide us with a solution.

What dogs offer so readily, of course, is precisely what physicians do not. Every year, our system equips us with more medicines to prescribe our patients yet less opportunity to sit down beside them and explain how they should be used. Each new administrative initiative brings us more tasks to complete and less time with which to complete them. Staffing cuts and bureaucratic demands force us to sprint through our days to accomplish the bare minimum of keeping our patients healthy, often leaving us unable to perform the critical task of simply slowing down to listen. As a result, we can find ourselves in the curious position of having saved our patients' lives, only to realize that they remain generally frustrated with their experience. More curiously, we understand that they are not necessarily wrong to feel this way.

And so, having found myself on the losing side of an end-of-shift tally to a puppy, I have come to appreciate that if I was ever going to make good on my original intention to "help people," it would not be by simply applying the skills I learned in medical school. Providing the correct medical treatments—even diligently saving lives—was not enough. I would also have to find opportunities to slow down, more fully embrace my patients' stories, and provide them with the respect they deserve. In other words, I would have to act a bit less like a doctor, and a bit more like my dog.

THREE

THE RELENTLESS MOMENTUM
OF SAVING A LIFE

We performed CPR for another couple of minutes, pumping more medications into the increasingly swollen, gray body with no change in status. A lifetime of memories, love and pain, joy and sorrow was now a hybrid of cool flesh and plastic tubes before us.

Me: You know what the husband's ETA is?
Paramedics: He followed us in a private vehicle [meaning his own car], so he should be here any minute.

Her body was not going to come back to life. We did our part and, at this point, would be comfortable in calling a time of death. But the idea that this woman's husband could rush in at any moment only to find us having moved on to other patients and appearing to ignore his loved one—him finding her dead, naked, and, worst of all, alone in an empty room—would be a tragedy separate from her death. It felt important to show him that we were with her and trying to help her. We may not have been able to change the outcome—we had no cures and no tricks up our sleeves—yet it felt important simply to be with his wife, demonstrating our concern when he arrived. Regardless, it was what my dog, Port, would do.

We stayed with the dead body and continued our futile efforts.

We were granted the flexibility of following our human instincts as there was little else to guide us. Even today, in the era of computerized medicine and protocolized decision making, there exists no definitive algorithm for the process of stopping a resuscitation attempt. It may come as a surprise, but the technical point at which we should cease our efforts and call a time of death is not clearly defined in the medical literature.

While many of our treatments—including when to *start* CPR—follow explicit formulas, the decision to *stop* CPR is curiously vague. Should we reach for a pulse and none is felt, for example, CPR is to be immediately and unambiguously begun. Similarly, when the rigid criteria for sepsis or a heart attack are met, we simply proceed with the treatments for those illnesses and get to work. The guidelines are crystal clear. But there remains no guideline for when to *stop* CPR— when to stop the attempt to resuscitate someone's life.

What this means is that, ultimately, there is no clear answer to the question, When is this dead person truly dead with absolutely no chance of recovery? Or, more practically, At what point do I stop trying to save them? This is a strange outlier in a world that is increasingly defined by metrics and flowcharts.

Early in my career, as I struggled to decide where I myself would draw the line, I often wondered why this might be the case. Why do we uniquely lack an answer to such a common and fundamentally important question? Perhaps, I thought, the sheer number of considerations that are required to be made so rapidly in these circumstances made it impossible to create such an algorithm. It is conceivable that no algorithm could capture the complexity of such a moment. For me as a doctor, the idea that there may still exist at least one area of medicine where physician judgment is valued more than a reflexic, robotic algorithm felt empowering.

Yet such an explanation felt more like an ego boost than an absolute truth. Indeed, many other algorithms tackle equally complex situations without difficulty. And so, part of me has always wondered whether the true reason for this is that we have collectively decided that opening the door to death by algorithm would be a bridge too far. Like the oasis of a nature preserve protected from the harsh geometry of the city, I wonder if we somehow appreciate that this one arena of medicine must be protected—that the final act of humanity must only be met by human decision making.

A resuscitation attempt carries so much momentum to act—to save a life—that stopping becomes surprisingly difficult. Most doctors are unwilling to stop even as futility becomes obvious. Even when we know someone is truly dead, it often feels that, as long as we keep trying, that person can remain among us. It is as if to stop trying is to give up on the *idea* of that person.

In these moments we are not merely tasked with trying to

save a patient's life, but also, through some mysterious trans-ference, it feels as if we take over their very will to live. When our patients are unconscious and unable to advocate for themselves, we become their survival drive. And so it feels as if stopping a resuscitation attempt is not mere acknowledgment of death, but, in fact, permission for it. It's as if we finally *allow* death when we say, "That's it. No more."

This idea of a physician taking over a patient's very nature is more than some personal delusion. It is, in fact, written into our very legal system. Incredibly, within the walls of a hospital, death is defined not by a person's final heartbeat, but by their physician's last chest compression. A person who dies in a hospital is not acknowledged as dead upon their last breath, as nature may dictate, but is dead when their *physician* declares agreement with nature's assessment.

If prior generations of physicians were said to have suffered from God complexes, then it may be because they actually codified their position as such.

As a result of this great pressure, it is understandable that most doctors err on the side of continuing their efforts far beyond any reasonable hope of recovery. After all, if someone is already dead, there is no possible way one could cause a worse outcome by continuing for an extra several minutes or so. Erring on the other end of the spectrum, however—stopping an attempt several minutes too early instead of several minutes too late—would keep most doctors up at night. So, it might be that we live with the ambiguity because there is simply too much at stake.

Whatever the reason, one of the most difficult decisions we need to make in medicine is left eerily ambiguous.

As a response, in an effort to simplify an outsized complexity, most doctors have created hard rules for themselves. "If the patient has been without a pulse for more than thirty minutes, unless they're a child, I stop immediately. I wouldn't have even taken your patient off the paramedic's cot," one doctor told me when I asked what he would have done in my situation. Yet another doctor told me: "I go for at least thirty minutes from *arrival* to the ER no matter what the paramedics say. Nothing against the paramedics; I just don't trust what *anyone* ever says." Impossibly, both opinions, while resulting in utterly dichotomous courses of action, are entirely appropriate.

We decided to stay with the dead body, continuing our treatment for just a few more moments until the husband arrived. It was reasonable medically to do so. And if doing so might help to provide comfort to this patient's husband by demonstrating our concern for her, it would be well worth the effort.

We could have called a time of death and simply told the husband that "both the paramedics and our team in the emergency room did everything we could, but we could not revive her." But having the patient's husband see the degree of effort and care directed toward his wife seemed more important than his hearing it. Extra resources would be used and other patients would have to wait longer to be seen, but here was an opportunity to make good on my premedical intention to "help people."

FOUR

THE ORCHESTRA AND ITS AUDIENCE OF ONE

Me: Okay, guys, Winston and Lewis are saying that the husband should be here any second, so if everyone is comfortable, let's continue for another minute or two. I think it would be better to continue for just a bit longer rather than stop now and have him walk in at that moment. Anyway, who knows, maybe we'll get a miracle?

There were nods of agreement.

CPR was administered. Epinephrine was pushed through the IV. Pulse checks were performed, never once bringing a hopeful flutter.

Finally, the patient's husband arrived. A nurse briefly explained what was happening—that his wife's heart had stopped beating and that we were doing what we could in order to undo that occurrence—and asked whether he preferred to join us inside, or stay outside and wait in a family room. Confirming his desire to be with his wife, he was ushered in.

Entering the bustling room, the husband was doing his best to remain calm and quiet. Nevertheless, his eyes revealed a frantic internal world. He stared at the inanimate body that was once his wife as he absorbed the scene around him.

While we understood the grim prognosis, the emergency room eradicates any ability to work in half-measures. In the emergency room, there is no such thing as slowing down or warming up. Like a binary language, there are only two modes of operation: all-in or not at all. And so, having decided that we were going to continue, we continued in full capacity.

I introduced myself.

> Me: Hello, sir, my name is Dr. Nahvi. As you know, your wife is not doing well and there is a lot going on right now. I want to talk to you at length and explain everything that's happening, but first I want to ask you a couple of quick questions just to make sure we're not missing anything—then we can talk more later on. Does that work?

He nodded.

Since I understood that each frenetic actor in front of me was playing a highly specific role in the pandemonium, the whole affair was fluent to me. I realized, however, that the scene must have looked utterly different to the patient's husband. Like watching a play in a foreign country without understanding the setting or the language, the entire display likely seemed chaotic. And, considering the stakes, probably terrifyingly so.

Standing by the patient's feet, leading the resuscitation, I surveyed the scene.

To my left, Alexandria, one of the kindest and hardest-working nurses I knew, was keeping track on a notepad of which medications were administered through which tubes, while simultaneously keeping time on a stopwatch. She was young but motherly in her care—I imagined she was responsible for the majority of the patients who left our emergency room happy. Her kindness, however, was not to be mistaken for timidity. When stakes were elevated and the circumstances required it, Alexandria took no prisoners. An aggressive advocate for her patients, she would stop at nothing to ensure they received whatever it was that they needed.

Looking up from her notebook to loudly shout "two minutes" at two-minute intervals in order to help us keep track of our progress, she must have seemed like a sort of strange, morbid referee.

Daris, another young nurse, had a firm affect that was backed up by a precocious skill set. One of the more talented nurses I have worked with, he often refused to do things that the doctors requested of him until he had the chance to look it up in a textbook or medical journal and independently confirm that it was the right thing to do. As one of those doctors, I gained confidence from his skepticism: if I had asked for something and Daris carried it out, it must have been the right thing to do.

Daris's role was to place intravenous lines and use the

various pumps and pressure bags to administer fluids, medications, and whatever other treatment might have been needed. Navigating the tangled mess of tubes that resembled jungle vines hanging from the canopy, he treated each patient like a military operation—he knew what he needed to do and would not let anything get in the way of his executing it. Reinforcing this image was his habit of offering a salute when confirming that he heard a request made of him.

Danny, an experienced physician assistant whom I would trust with my own life, was another essential member of the team. His role was to examine the patient and report his findings to the team. He hovered around the patient's body like an unshakable mosquito. Finding something to inspect and analyze, he would get close to our patient, placing a stethoscope on her chest or shining a penlight in her eyes. Satisfied with what he found, he would step back once more before buzzing over to another part of her body.

A hardworking and affable man, Danny felt like some sort of master of the mystic arts. He pursued strange diagnoses based on hunches that often turned out to be correct.

During our shifts, Danny would often come to me saying things like, "I think we should get a CT scan of this girl's head—she's young and healthy and probably just has the flu so there's no obvious indication to do it—but for *some reason* I'm worried about her. She's complaining of a headache and it just doesn't seem to be a normal type of headache for the flu. I just *feel* like there might be something else going on." With time I learned that it would take either an extraordinarily bold or an extraordinarily dumb physician to override one of

Danny's hunches. His instinct tested our hierarchy. As a physician assistant, he technically had to run things by me, but I often had little to add to the plans he had already come up with. "Sounds great, I think you're right, let's do it" was the most common response I had to whatever it was he suggested.

Examining the dead patient before us, Danny would help us look for clues that could identify a possible cause of death that we could then go on to treat, and, ideally, reverse. There was nobody better suited for the job.[1]

At the back of the room, observing everything like a cold and calculating headmaster, stood Ms. Summer, one of the supervising nurses. She was tall in height but short in demeanor. She was sometimes biting in her criticism and had a stern disposition. Over time, however, I had spied her privately being so overwhelmingly warm and caring to enough people and on enough occasions that I came to understand that her projected disposition was merely a facade. Her hard shell shielded her true character of gentle affection.

Very likely, as an African American woman in a leadership position, Ms. Summer needed her facade. Her job was to make sure everything was in order—from the supplies we needed to have available, to staff showing up on time and performing their jobs diligently. If the emergency room was to function, it was essential that Ms. Summer's orders be followed. Respect was critical. About a decade her junior, I was deferential to her. I understood that should I ever need anything within the walls of the hospital, she had the power to make things happen.

Our three patient care technicians, Rodrigo, Simon, and

Armando, were the kinetic energy of the scene. They were either actively performing chest compressions to allow our patient's heart to pump, squeezing a self-inflating bag in order to send air through her lungs, or waiting on deck to take over one of those two jobs. Collectively they were performing the job that our patient's young body was failing to do for itself. Like the Queen's Guards, the three men diligently cycled through their roles in predetermined intervals so as to ensure that they would not tire out.

Witnessing Rodrigo, Simon, and Armando perform their work allows one to truly appreciate the wonder of the human body. We live our entire lives with our hearts and lungs continuously beating and breathing, barely aware of the constant mechanics that allow for our very survival. Yet when our organs have quit and others attempt to replicate their intrinsic functions from the outside, it is impossible to ignore the tremendous work our organs have been doing all along. In order to pump our patient's heart after it had quit beating and to inflate her lungs after they failed to inspire, three grown men would have to drip with sweat and heave with breathlessness.

Beyond acting as surrogates for her body's failed organs, Rodrigo, Simon, and Armando also served as our patient's medication delivery system. While it was Daris who measured our syringes and injected their contents into our patient's arm, those medications would go nowhere were it not for the chest compressions that Rodrigo, Simon, and Armando were providing. When one's heart fails to pump, one's blood ceases to flow, causing our body's fluids and the medications dissolved in them to lie stagnant. And so, beyond merely providing oxygen to our patient's brain, Rodrigo, Simon, and Armando's efforts allowed our medications to course through her veins.

Each in their fifties, the three men were older than the typical member of the overnight shift. Despite having plenty of opportunity to work more agreeable schedules, they nevertheless stuck with the graveyard shift. I suspected that they simply wanted to do their job without the invasive oversight of hospital administration judging their every move. They prized their freedom—it was only when the hospital's business administrators left their offices for the day that Rodrigo, Simon, and Armando would begin to show up for their shift. The three of them were genuinely good friends, and seeing them together at work—privately sharing a laugh, a secret, or a meal—always brought a smile to my face.

Daniela, our scribe, was the youngest member of our team. She was off to the side diligently taking notes on the scene unfolding before us. She recorded our conversation with the paramedics, our rapport among ourselves, what quantities of medications we administered and the times at which we did so, as well as the physical findings we would note aloud. Ultimately, she would organize this information into a document that would become our patient's medical, legal, and—due to the realities of our system—financial record.

While technically on the ground floor of our team's medical hierarchy, Daniela became a friend of mine by rejecting the very notion of such a hierarchy. Rebuffing hospital decorum, she refused to call me "Dr. Nahvi," instead referring to me by my first name from the day we were introduced. I admired her for exerting her independence, and we bonded over our shared distaste for all things staid and stuffy.

Daniela cared for our patients above all. Her priorities were not well rounded, and I respected her tremendously for it. She often skirted the actual responsibilities of her job in order to do the right thing. When she went missing, I knew I could find her in a patient room, quietly helping a homeless patient change his socks or cutting the food on an elderly patient's dinner tray into small pieces so they could eat it more comfortably. She was often in trouble with her supervisors, who reprimanded her for going rogue by order of her moral compass. I could not help but think that if we were all so bold—if we all did the right thing despite the world's expectations— the world would be a much better place. Through her actions, Daniela advocated for a less efficient, but more caring, society. I admired her for it—Daniela, bad at her job, was an expert at life.

Finally, leading the resuscitation attempt, I stood at the foot of the patient's bed like a conductor of a grim orchestra or some sort of mission control. Information came from every corner. "Pupils are fixed and unresponsive to light," Danny offered from the head of the patient's bed, beaming a penlight into her eyes. "The IV in the left antecube isn't working anymore," Daris, now off to the side, announced. "We're going to be due for another round of epi and a pulse check in fifteen seconds," said Alexandria, looking up from her scorecard. "It looks like the ET tube needs to be suctioned," Rodrigo noted in the middle of his chest compressions.

"Um, sorry to interrupt, Dr. Nahvi, I know you guys are

busy, but your patient in room twelve just started complaining of shortness of breath and their oxygen is actually a little low," a nurse informed us from the doorway, bringing unwelcome news from the outside world.

My task was to filter this information, decide on a course of action, and clearly communicate that plan with our team. I took care to slow down my racing thoughts in order to process all the information coming my way and create a plan. Our actions have to be quick—but in order to work effectively, our thought processes need to remain slow and deliberate.

"Slow is smooth. Smooth is fast. Slow is fast," a mentor I deeply admired had once taught me. I processed the information coming my way, thought through the possible courses of action, weighed the potential risks and benefits of each one as well as their likelihood of occurring, and then, ultimately, created a strategy. Upon doing so, I communicated that strategy to my team for its execution.

As in all high-stakes circumstances, our language became sharper and more precise. Every observation and request is directed to a specific person. That person then clearly verifies that they heard the request and affirms that they will act on it. We stop all unnecessary communication. Everything that is said, however, is said twice.

"Got it, Danny, that's no good about the pupils. I'm going to stay here, but can you please step out to go check on that patient with shortness of breath in room twelve and let me know what's going on? And no worries, Daris, we have an eighteen-gauge IV working great on the right side for now.

Let's get ready for another round of epi and pulse check but then after that could we please try to get another working IV on the left side? If we can't get one we can always consider an IO in the tibia, but I don't think it'll be necessary. And thanks for the heads up, Rodrigo, could you and Ms. Summer please work on suctioning the ET tube?"[2]

The responses echoed back: "Okay, I am going to step out of the room and check up on that patient in room twelve," from Danny. "You got it, epi coming right up and then I'll get another IV going on the left side," from Daris, accompanied by a salute. "No problem, I'll suction the tube," Rodrigo confirmed to the group.

The patient's husband stood behind me, soaking in the scene.

FIVE

A DESPERATE SEARCH FOR CLUES

I have learned that most people do not understand the gravity of a resuscitation attempt in real time. As a result, their reactions are often painful to watch. In medicine, "pulseless," "CPR," and "coding" all effectively mean "dead." These words are only uttered once the heart has already ceased to function properly. As discussed, in rare instances, we can get a heart to successfully beat once again, but when any of these words are uttered, the prognosis is almost always bleak.

Nevertheless, in the middle of the resuscitation of a pulseless patient, some family members look to our words with optimism. Mistaking our status updates for progress, their eyes light up when we speak. Unfamiliar with the circumstances they have suddenly been thrust into, they look to us for signs of hope when there are none. The disconnect between the reality of our words and what they hope them to mean can be difficult to bridge.

I have witnessed family members hold their loved one's cold hands and attempt to coach them back to life. "C'mon, beat this! You can do it! You're a fighter!" they might yell, as if their loved one's failed heart was caused by insufficient drive and determination. Doggedly optimistic, these people are driven by unrealistic expectations. As we watch them make their pleas, we know that their innocence to the situation often leads to a more painful, crashing realization down the line.

Feeling helpless in the chaos, many family members panic and interrupt, excitedly offering us tidbits of varied information. "Oh! I forgot to tell you!" they might interject, "She ate leftover pizza this morning for breakfast when she woke up and she said that it tasted funny." Or, alternatively, "Just so you know, she had a major back surgery twelve years ago and has had a lot of back pain ever since."

It is a bit like recalling last year's weather in California as we try to predict today's forecast in New York. These bits of data may be completely true, but they are completely unrelated. They are clues for a different puzzle.

Nevertheless, while these interruptions may be functionally irrelevant, we do not dismiss them. We understand that they are nothing more than manifestations of desperation—loved ones grasping for hope in their most powerless moment. Unwilling to coldly wave them off, we instead express appreciation for these bits of irrelevant data.

Unaffected by Hollywood's version of this type of situation, we know the true odds in front of us. And so, in an attempt to save *something*, we do our best to empower these family members. At the very least, we hope, we can help these family members walk away with the confidence that they did everything they could to help their loved one.

We appreciate their efforts and we nod our heads knowingly. "Ah, cold pizza for breakfast? Okay, thanks very much. Did anything else happen this morning?" we might ask.

Unlike many other family members, however, this patient's husband remained still and silent. His eyes did not light up. He did not nervously pace around the room, make pleas to his wife, or interject with any information.

Instead, he would react with a whimper every time "no pulse" was announced after a pulse check. Rather than indulge a sense of false optimism, he would put his head back between his hands with every "resume CPR" that we called out. He remained silent in his own internal universe. He simply stared at his wife and absorbed the scene in front of him. It was evident that he had no illusions about what was occurring. His eyes showed little optimism. Each minute that went by seemed to fill him with more agony. He knew, it seemed, that his wife had died, and that the odds were slim.

While his reaction was perhaps more accurate than that of other family members, it was not any easier to watch. Instead, his presence was difficult to absorb precisely because he seemed to understand so much. It was clear that he was experiencing the gravity of the moment as we were, in real time.

I went over to him to probe him for answers. I looked for any clue that could help explain what it was that brought his young wife to her death.

Me: Our friends with EMS told me that your wife didn't have any medical problems. Is that accurate?

The patient's husband nodded. "Yeah, she was totally healthy."

Me: And they said she was complaining only of some abdominal pain and some chest pain throughout the day until she collapsed and passed out? Was there anything else bothering her? Maybe earlier today? Earlier this week?

Husband (this time with a tear): Nope, that's it. She was complaining of stomach pain for about two days, but it wasn't so bad until today. Today it got worse and she also developed some chest pain, too, so that's why we called 911. She was also feeling a little short of breath, I guess, but really, it was the belly pain that was bothering her. That was the main thing that she was complaining about.

I thought about my desire to continue our efforts so that this man could witness his wife's death and the care and attention she received.

Previous generations of doctors, following the same instinct of care, would do just the opposite. Rather than take a few extra steps to ensure that a family member could be present as their loved one died, they would instead rush to escort family members outside the room to make sure they would not be there as it happened. These physicians believed they were protecting family members from seeing their loved one under such compromised circumstances. It was as if they believed civilized society was too fragile to witness the ugliness of death. I have always found the idea that people should be protected from their family member's reality troublesome, however well intentioned. More than anyone else, I believe, it is they who *should* be in the room, spending their last moments with their loved ones.

Recent research has validated this idea.[1] A good body of evidence exists to support the idea that, far from traumatizing them further, witnessing the process of their loved one's death actually gives family members closure. Staying in the room as a loved one dies eliminates mystery and provides insight. It provides confidence that significant efforts were made to save their loved one. Ultimately, we now know that family members who are part of a failed resuscitation attempt go on to have a less difficult grieving process than those who are unable to witness the process. This truth would be widely recognized during the Covid-19 pandemic, when so many people around the world were denied the opportunity to be with their loved ones as they died in isolation.

A "less difficult grieving process," however, does not mean an easy one.

Having family members in the room, hearing them wail and scream, and seeing them double over in anguish beside their loved one's body removes death from our sterile clinical environment and places it squarely into a messy emotional one. Seeing this man silently shed tears and release an occasional whimper forced us to see his wife not as a pulseless patient requiring Advanced Cardiovascular Life Support (ACLS), but as the dead wife of a newly widowed husband.

I have come to appreciate, then, that previous generations of doctors were not whisking family members away only in order to protect them. Very likely they were also doing so in order to protect themselves.

> Me: Is there anything else that you feel is important for us to know? To be honest, as of right now, it's not perfectly clear to me what the cause of all this was— can you think of anything else that might help us identify what might have happened? Any recent—

Alexandria interrupted, dutifully refereeing our progress: "Two minutes!" she shouted. I interrupted my conversation with the husband and turned back toward the team.

> Me: Okay, guys, let's hold compressions and do a pulse check. Who's up next for compressions? . . . I don't feel a pulse, does anyone feel a pulse? . . . No? . . . Okay, no pulse then; please resume compressions.

I turned back to the husband. "Sorry. Anything else that could help us identify a cause for all this? Any recent illnesses? Any drug use? Could she be pregnant by any chance? Any recent long flights or history of blood clots or anything?[2]

> Husband: Well, we recently flew back from Florida for vacation last week, but no, she was fine there, we had a

great time. And no, no illnesses and no history of blood clots and definitely no other drugs or anything. She's a totally normal person. And no, she's not pregnant. We tried for years, but we were never able to get pregnant.

Me: Okay, that is super helpful, thank you so much. I'm going to give my attention back to the team now. You are welcome to stay in the room if you'd like but you certainly don't have to if you prefer to wait outside.

The husband neither moved nor said a word. Whether by conscious decision or from being frozen by the avalanche of emotions he was experiencing, he opted to stay in the room.

Over a decade ago, I chose to specialize in emergency medicine thinking that "if bad things—heart attacks, strokes, shootings, stabbings—are happening, I might as well be the one to be there and take care of them when they do."

Years later, however, that rationale is tested whenever I am actually dealing with one of those "bad things." In those moments, I am not rationalizing that "at least I'm helping" or "it would still be happening whether I were here or not." Instead, some deeply primitive part of my brain becomes a child throwing a tantrum. "I hate that any of this is happening at all!" it screams. Uselessly, I perseverate on the impossible. Knowing that I could not save this patient, I simply wanted to go back in time and undo her death.

It is incredible how one can simultaneously carry such wildly contrasting trains of thoughts in their mind. On one hand, building off terabytes of evidence-based medicine, evidence created from decades of randomized controlled trials and meta-analyses, my mind methodically churned through all the possible reversible causes of death and their likelihoods. On the other hand, feeling equally at home in my brain was a series of functionally useless, crude emotional wails.

Me: Just so you fully understand, the situation is very bad, your wife is unresponsive and without a pulse, so right now she is technically not alive and our efforts and the efforts of the paramedics haven't been able to turn things around so far. We haven't had any good signs yet, and as time goes on, it's looking more and more unlikely that we will be able to change that.

The patient's husband remained still. He stood in the back of the room, expressing his preference to remain with his wife and be a part of her death.

SIX

TO RECALIBRATE A HUMAN BEING

After several more moments—the clinical status of our patient unchanged, but the husband now present—I revisited the idea of stopping our efforts with my team.

> Me: Okay, everyone, just to recap, we have a forty-three-year-old female, healthy, no past medical problems, with a recent return flight from Florida last week who was complaining of abdominal pain and chest pain and then shortness of breath. When the paramedics arrived she appeared well but then collapsed and was pulseless. ACLS was performed for over thirty minutes in the field and another ten minutes or so here in the emergency room. We haven't been able to get a pulse back at any point, her end-tidal CO_2 never got above ten, and her bedside ECHO shows no cardiac activity. Glucose was normal, we have no reason to suspect

any potassium issues, and she's already intubated, which would have taken care of hypoxia as a cause, however unlikely that would have been.[1] We have a low concern for ACS[2] causing any of this. I know she had abdominal pain and her recent flight was too short to technically be a true risk factor so it doesn't totally fit, but my highest concern is still for a pulmonary embolism.[3] That said, she has already been down and pulseless for a total of over forty minutes now and I cannot think of anything we could give her or do for her that would change the ultimate outcome. Please let me know if I'm missing anything or if anyone has any ideas. Otherwise, if everyone is on the same page, I think it is time to stop our resuscitation and call a time of death.

The room remained largely quiet. Murmurs of muted agreement came from various members of the team.

Me: Okay, if anyone has any additional thoughts, please speak up now.

I secretly hoped someone would interject with a plan. Perhaps they would inform me of a new death-reserving medication that I had not yet read about.

Instead, nobody said a word. The only response I received was a muttering chorus of murmured dejection. While unintelligible, it was the unmistakable sound of disappointment.

Me: Okay, then, Armando, please stop the chest
compressions. Great job, everyone. Time of death:
6:27 a.m.

Medicine often thrusts us into strange situations that can sometimes feel as if they are pulled from an entirely different reality. The sheer oddness of some of these situations forces us to adopt new, often bizarre, standards.

I told my team they did a "great job," and I meant it. Everyone performed their job skillfully, and we worked diligently and efficiently. Yet we had no tangible success. It was, by any sane account, a failure. The woman remained dead and we did nothing to change her situation. At no point did we even briefly get a pulse back only to lose it again later—the entirety of our efforts could not even afford her miserable heart just a few extra ticks.

I remember a patient I helped to care for once when I was in medical school. I was rotating through the intensive care unit, treating a man who was the victim of a violent assault. His assault had caused him to bleed inside his skull, beside his brain. He had fractured several bones in his neck, causing them to impinge on his spinal cord. He had lost his ability to control his arms, his legs, and even his bowels.

Comatose, he lay in the intensive care unit—one tube breathing for him, another tube feeding him. An entire army of nurses and patient technicians was charged with the sole task of shifting his flaccid body to a new position every two hours. They came in teams and dutifully performed their mission: on to his right side at noon, over to his back at two. He was to be turned all the way to his left side at four, before restarting the cycle and bringing him back to his right side at six. Through day and night this patient was constantly being moved and yet, in so many ways, he was going nowhere at all. All of this human labor was being expended just so the weight of his body did not break down his flesh, creating painful pressure ulcerations that could lead to dangerous or even deadly infections.

His body had become a rotisserie chicken, continually needing to be rotated in order to prevent any one part of it from becoming too damaged. His personhood had been reduced so that the simplest law of physics was now his enemy. His MRI results suggested a poor prognosis. He would certainly never walk, and it was unlikely that he would ever be able to speak. Chances were, in fact, that he would never even recognize his family again.

Yet each day his family would come in to check on him, and each day the attending physician would check in with them to note whatever progress might have been made. I remember the family meeting on the day that he spontaneously opened his eyes.

"Well, we have some good news for you today," the attending physician said in a neutral tone. "He made some progress and was able to open his eyes on his own today."

What kind of sadistic madness is this? I remember thinking to myself as I listened in on the conversation. I remember feeling disgusted, with an urgent desire to escape the room. I thought of excusing myself to the restroom just so I could leave.

My disgust, of course, was not directed toward any specific person. I was not at all mad at the physician and I was certainly not upset that the patient had opened his eyes. After all, it *was* progress in the most literal sense of the word: he had been unable to open his eyes yesterday, and today he was able to.

Rather, I was disgusted at such a dismal recalibration of a human being, at how heartbreakingly low our standards for a man had fallen. From my inexperienced point of view, that a man who could not recognize his wife from a wall had merely opened his eyes was not a cause for celebration. His life had been smashed. Whether his eyes could open or whether they would remain shut while he lay there unable to control his arms, legs, or basic bodily functions seemed to me of little significance. If anything, I thought, celebrating that most pitiful of accomplishments only highlighted how much was lost.

But after hearing the news, the family smiled back at the doctor, to my surprise. To be certain, they had no false optimism—the attending physician had gone on to tell them plainly that the fact that he opened his eyes did not change the prognosis that he would likely never walk, eat, or even recognize them again.

Nevertheless, they were pleased. However I perceived the information, the patient's family, it seemed, was appreciative. That their father could now open his eyes—regardless of whether he actually saw anything when he did so—seemed to matter to them. And that it mattered to them mattered to me.

I remember being forced to rethink my own reaction. The entire family had experienced a sudden and tumultuous shock—a devastating turbulence after which nothing would ever be the same. Their life was now split into two distinct phases: 1) Pre–dad's assault and 2) Post–dad's assault.

The reality was that their father was not dead, but was permanently changed. By necessity of their new circumstance, they *had* to undergo a recalibration. They had to redefine, for themselves, the very definition of success and failure. They would have to decide from scratch what was, and what was not, a cause for celebration. They needed a new set of standards. Perhaps they may have now thought, when they looked at him, at least they could look into his eyes.

And so, slowly, after years of training and becoming more and more familiar with so many dreadfully strange situations—after so many rethinkings of what constituted horror and what constituted relief—I came to appreciate this ability to recalibrate. I came to understand that everything was entirely relative, and that no sign, symptom, or action meant anything without its broader context. I came to appreciate the inherently strange circumstances of my work.

Indeed, on our current day, despite our undeniably dismal outcome of death, our team *did* do great work. They functioned smoothly and quickly. Everybody knew their roles and performed at the highest possible level. The chest compressions were strong and reliable; medications were administered at the appropriate intervals. Every relevant action was considered and executed without hesitation or delay. In a slightly different scenario—a different patient or a different set of circumstances, perhaps—this type of expert-level performance *could* have resurrected the dead.

Our team did great work and they deserved to know it. Strange as it may be to say, it was appropriate to have said it. And so, in the twisted culture of medicine, there is nothing incongruent about telling one's team they did "great work" as a dead body lies before them. For the prospect of future patients who might be saved by such efforts and for my team's own morale, it was only right that they were acknowledged.

Nevertheless, I wondered what the husband, without the context of experiences that we have had, might have thought. I wondered whether he found my phrasing insulting or, perhaps, whether he found it comforting. On one hand, it must be difficult to hear my team complimented on our collective failure. It is not unreasonable that the husband might become offended or angry to see others get a collective pat on the back as his wife lay dead before them. On the other hand, it might have instilled in him some confidence that there were no mistakes or missed opportunities. After all, hearing that the team caring for his wife did a great job also meant that everything that could have been done for her, was.

Nevertheless, I have learned that there is no way to predict how someone might internalize and respond to hearing such things. I remember, during my first year of residency training, evaluating a patient who had come to the emergency room because of a simple allergic rash. I inspected it, brushing my hand over her skin and assessing it for the raised hives that are a classic marker of an allergic reaction. Noting my gloved hands, she became offended. "What am I? Diseased? It's not contagious, it's an allergic reaction. You have to put gloves on to touch me?" she complained.

Early in my training and deeply sensitive to such complaints, I internalized the scolding. A respected mentor from medicine's old school even weighed in. "Don't forget the power of touch," he told me. "Washed hands are just as clean as gloved ones. Using your bare hands demonstrates a certain solidarity with your patients—it shows them that since you're not afraid of them, they should not be afraid of their illness, either."

I was convinced. Months later, I evaluated another patient for a nearly identical complaint. Washing my hands with soap and water and evaluating the rash on his upper arm without any gloves, I received another rebuke.

While our real-time interaction was unremarkable, I was told weeks later that the hospital had received a written complaint. "The doctor who examined me didn't even put gloves on when he touched my rash. It was disgusting. What kind of hospital is this?" the patient had written. This time, a different mentor weighed in: "I'd just wear the gloves. You never know what a patient might have and it's always good to protect yourself." It felt as if I were damned no matter which action I took.

Nevertheless, it was an important lesson.

While we may be presented with the same stimuli, we are all informed by wildly different life experiences, personalities, and mental models of how the world works. There are no obvious answers. What fits best for one person might not work for others. The ways in which we understand and react to the world are infinitely layered and complex. Very simply, we can try to be sensitive to how others may perceive us, but we can never know what is going on in someone else's mind. We may never understand how others will react to what we say or do.

But we cannot let this paralyze us. Ultimately, we must do what we think to be right.

I turned around to face the husband, who was now seated behind me, tears still in his eyes. I began to speak. "I'm very sorry." After a long pause, I continued. "How about we sit down and talk and go over everything that's happened?"

"Sure. What are the next steps?" the husband asked me. "Do I call a funeral home? Is there paperwork to fill out? What should I do?"

Despite the understandings I claim to have developed, I never cease to be surprised that so many people's first reaction to the death of their loved ones is to ask about protocol.

Perhaps focusing on the more pedestrian details surrounding death is a sort of coping mechanism. Perhaps by focusing on paperwork, the funeral home—anything else—families can delay comprehending the fact that their loved one has actually died. Perhaps it is an effort to exert control over a situation that nobody can truly control. Filling out a mindless form or making a decision about a funeral home probably allows one to re-exert control over their environment rather than simply be forced into reacting to it. Or, perhaps, our lives are often so task-oriented that, in a way, pursuing yet another task can be something of a comfort. *If I act normally, things will be normal.*

Irrationally, I am offended at the notion of dealing with paperwork so soon after a death. My brain reflexively thinks, *This is no time to be thinking about the bureaucrats! Someone has just died!*

Then I immediately snap back and remember that the person making the comment is the one closest to the deceased.

That person—not me—is the only one with any right to actual offense. I remind myself that I have not had the experiences they have had, that there is no way that I could put myself in their place. If they feel it is appropriate to focus on the paper-work, then it is appropriate to focus on the paperwork.

Regardless, it never ceases to be jarring: the adrenaline and high emotion of death, and then a calm discussion of adminis-trative forms to be filled out. I have witnessed many different reactions—anger, disbelief, acceptance, even relief—yet the grieving process nevertheless remains mysterious to me.

> **Me:** For now, there is nothing that needs to be done other
> than what you feel that you need to do. We can give
> you as much time as you'd like. There will be some
> paperwork to fill out—our clerk Benny has it all at his
> desk, but we can worry about all that later, or we could
> do it now if you want. We should also sit down and
> talk to discuss everything, but you let me know when
> you're ready for that. In the meanwhile I only have one
> suggestion: it might be a good idea to call some family
> or friends to come be with you at this time as well.
> Is there anyone you might want me to call on your
> behalf? Of course, that is up to you too.
> **Husband:** Okay. Thanks. Can I have a minute here alone
> with her first, and then we can talk?
> **Me:** Of course.

I stepped out of the room.

SEVEN

GUNSHOT WOUNDS, FORK SWALLOWERS, AND THE TRUTH

As the patient's husband paused to collect his thoughts, I thought about how rarely we, the treatment team, take that time for ourselves. We are familiar with death, yet we avoid talking about it. Like a passenger one regularly sees on their morning commute but has never spoken with, death is simultaneously a familiar face and a distant stranger.

Upon learning that I am an emergency medicine doctor, people often ask how I deal with encountering death. "It must be stressful. How do you do it?"

It is a difficult question to answer. I usually shrug it off. "You get used to it," I say.

That is a lie. You don't get used to it.

I have been intimately involved in a wide variety of deaths. I have experienced grandparents dying of cancer and heart disease and have seen children die of illnesses and injury. I have filled out the morbid paperwork required after a successful suicide attempt. I have informed a pair of French tourists that the precarious selfie they warned their daughter not to take would be the last picture they would have of her. I have told the intoxicated driver of a rollover car crash that he would be spending the remainder of spring break—and beyond— without his best friend. I have never gotten used to any of it.

Instead, I often feel the need to change the subject. Asked about the misfortune of death, I deflect to a story about a patient who came in seeking assistance in removing a Magic Marker from his rectum. Asked about the misery death leaves in its wake, I steer the conversation toward a prisoner who learned to swallow forks in order to get transferred out of his jail cell and into the infirmary. Asked about death itself, I do not tell about the gunshot victims who died, but about the rare one who survived. I describe the miracles performed by our trauma surgeons as they fillet a young man's thorax wide open, massage his heart out of his chest cavity, sew up the hole that the bullet made as it plowed through the chambers of his heart, and ultimately place his heart, beating on its own once more, back inside his chest.

My lies and my deflections are not an effort to hide some other, hidden truth. There is no secret that I prefer to keep to myself. Nor am I protecting my audience from stories that I assume they would prefer not to hear. The reality is that I demur simply because I do not know what else to say.

I know that I am not alone in having failed to properly address the many dire situations we face in medicine. In fact, most of the doctors and nurses I know have never formally confronted this fundamental aspect of our jobs. The truth is that, as a whole, we rarely tell our stories to anyone. We study death academically, but in no part of our training do we take a step back and ask, "What do these deaths mean to us? How do they impact us and our world? What do I do now, having been intimately involved in the death of this stranger?"

Once, I arrived at work only to make my way through a waiting room filled with about two dozen distraught individuals. Along with their makeup and styled hair, they were outfitted in their finest suits and dresses. A coworker told me that hours prior to my arrival on shift, he had pronounced the death of a twenty-four-year-old woman, on her wedding day. She had collapsed in the middle of her wedding reception while dancing with her new husband. She had arrived to the emergency room in cardiac arrest, still in her wedding gown. Months away from his own wedding himself, my colleague told me how the symbolism of this torn wedding dress—the white gown sheared into pieces as a result of our team's efforts to access her arteries and veins—troubled him and he could not shake the image. He told me how he was planning to leave through a back door when making his way home so he would not have to face the weeping wedding party in our waiting room.

After telling me about his experience, this coworker simply shrugged his shoulders and walked away. "Jeez, what can you do? It's just crazy," he said as he went on to see his subsequent patients.

Another friend, an obstetrician colleague, once told me of a patient who died unexpectedly of a blood clot in her lungs hours after giving birth to her first baby. Prior to her patient's sudden death, this physician noted how both husband and wife would light up with eagerness in their eyes when they would discuss their plans together as a new family. That future taken from them in an instant, my friend explicitly noted how this husband was now destined to celebrate each of his newborn baby's birthdays in the shadow of his wife's death. She remarked on how impossibly difficult it must be for this newborn child to grow up knowing that each birthday was also an anniversary of the death of her mother.

"I don't know, it's just tough," was ultimately all this friend was able to muster after she described her harrowing scenario.

I once watched a third colleague lead a failed resuscitation of a six-month-old infant. The child was left with his mother's boyfriend for several hours while she was at work. Unable to get the baby to stop crying, the boyfriend shook the baby, irreversibly silencing him. Further convoluting matters, the baby's mother happened to work as a pediatrician herself. She was called at her office in the middle of her workday while caring for other children, in order to come to the emergency room so that she could be informed that her own child had been killed by her boyfriend.

I remember watching the physician who delivered the news, a parent herself, silently walk out of the room after speaking with the patient's mother and the New York City police officers who had become involved in the case. Quietly and without expressing any outward emotion, she simply sat down at her computer terminal, logged into her email account, and began scrolling through her emails.

It is not that these doctors were callous or unaffected by these scenarios. I know all of these physicians personally and am certain that they were all deeply affected by the encounters they had had. It is, very simply, that we somehow lack the capacity to truly process and discuss these events.

These tragedies are so profound that they exist beyond our normal ability to understand and communicate them. It would be like someone who has only seen flatlands and prairies trying to fathom the size and scale of Mount Everest. As much as that person may claim to understand, the truth is that it is hard for one to truly wrap one's head around such scale. Unable to fully grasp their experience, it is more difficult still to explain it to others. Adjectives and hyperbole can take one only so far. At a certain point, language itself fails us.

These circumstances feel bigger than our ability to communicate them. Feeling something so powerfully, yet finding oneself unable to communicate the depth of that feeling, can be deflating. We are left feeling powerless. So, unable to adequately communicate our experiences, we often stop trying to communicate them altogether. Counterintuitively, it is the very magnitude of their importance that might be the cause of our failure to address them.

"Nobody's ever really going to 'get it' unless they are a part of it," I have heard older physicians tell young doctors as they mentor them with particularly myopic advice. "They can't. It's all just too crazy."

We are left with a strange paradox: the very profession that knowingly puts us inside the arena with death simultaneously lacks any framework to enable us to engage with it in a meaningful way. We spend all day listening to stories, but never quite learn how to tell them.

As a result, the reality of what takes place after a death in a hospital is strikingly ordinary.

In the emergency room, when a death occurs, after the time of death is announced, the inertia in the room dampens, the adrenaline slowly returns to baseline, and the team caring for the patient makes knowing eye contact. We bow our heads, absorb the futility of our collective efforts, pull the curtains closed behind us, and walk out of the room to pick up where we left off.

That brief moment of knowing eye contact is the full extent of the grieving process. There is no discussion; there is no ceremony. There is not even a pause in our workflow. Our emergency rooms understaffed and our waiting rooms overcrowded, the demands of myriad other ill and injured patients waiting to be seen prevent us from even slowing down. The acknowledgment of the end of a life is no more than a brief and somber glance. The entire affair is striking in its inadequacy.

I thought back to the first time I came across a dead patient in the emergency room. I was a medical student and had just arrived at the beginning of my shift. We reviewed our patients as a group in order that the previous team, preparing to go home, could transfer their responsibilities over to us. As we did this, we skipped one patient bed. The curtains were closed. The incoming physician asked about the omission. It was then that I first heard the term "expired" used in reference to a human being.

"Oh, don't worry about him. I'll take care of everything before I leave. That patient expired about an hour ago," the outgoing doctor said. His tone was understandably muted and his demeanor was respectful. Yet I was struck by the way he referred to a human being with a term more often used to describe a gallon of milk or a coupon code.

I noted how this physician drew the curtain tighter to more thoroughly hide the body as we rounded, and I noted how he lowered his eyes and hushed his voice when he spoke of the man's "expiration." I noted that he still smiled as he spoke with his other patients, so as to not let them in on his secret. I noted that he told us "not to worry" about the dead patient, not because of anything related to the tragedy of his death, but because he would be taking care of the paperwork that accompanied it. I noted that he did not linger or dwell on the case—that the entirety of his acknowledgment of the death of a human being lasted no more than four or five seconds.

Seeing this physician note that a person had died with about the same degree of urgency that someone might note that it had stopped raining outside, or that traffic on the expressway was heavier than usual, sent its own powerful signal. By the end of that day, the first day my small cohort of medical students had heard the word "expired" in reference to a human being, we had all begun parroting the new language as if we had been using it our whole lives. "Did you ever figure out what the expired patient expired from?" we would ask one another. Ignoring our human instincts, we looked to our superiors and believed this cold, dissociating language was not only normal, but correct.

It is not clear to me why, as a professional culture, we in medicine have so summarily failed to interact meaningfully with death. One might be forgiven for wanting to believe that the type of projected indifference we put forth is simply a necessary survival tactic. Perhaps, one might argue, doctors and nurses develop this clinical dissociation in order that we not become too overwhelmed. After all, were we to become too invested in every tragic outcome we witness in the emergency room, we might become paralyzed to the point of inaction.

Yet such an explanation feels shortsighted. It takes little more than a brief analysis to realize that it cannot possibly be true. Avoiding a topic does not make it go away. *Pretending* not to be impacted by death does not *make* one unaffected by it. We do not naturally build immunity against the effects of death, any more than we build immunity against love or any other powerful emotion. The effects of these profound emotions do not diminish with repetition; they compound.

So, if anyone seriously believes that ignoring our reality is our best coping mechanism, I fear that they have miscalculated. If one remains unconvinced, I would point them to the alarmingly high rates of depersonalization, burnout, mental illness, and even suicide we see in medicine today.

I do not believe our medical culture has purposefully created our ill-fated ethos. I do not believe that any doctor or nurse has ever consciously thought that the best way to deal with these troubling emotions is to close oneself off to them. I do not believe that we have avoided exploring our experiences and telling our stories by design.

Common things being common, I believe our collective failure to interact meaningfully with these experiences is the result of a failure just like any other human failure. More likely, we fail to speak about our experiences for the same reason that so many people fail to save enough money for retirement or never get around to losing the extra ten pounds they always tell themselves they are going to lose: We *know* that we need to do better, but we don't get around to doing the hard and uncomfortable work needed to do it.

As a result, we claim that "nobody will ever understand" the very thing that we will all, one day, experience. We claim that the most constant and fundamental of human experiences is "too crazy" for others to comprehend. We muster little more than awkward gazes, nods of mutual understanding, and knowing eye contact. And we scroll through our emails, failing to reflect and engage with our world in the way that we must.

EIGHT

"ISN'T EVERYTHING IN THE EMERGENCY ROOM AN EMERGENCY?"

Walking out of a room where a patient has died, where stakes were high and the energy in the air matched it, one immediately reenters the world of the living. Like a new father heading back to his job after a brief paternity leave, we return to our work pretending things remained just as they were before—although secretly, we understand that everything has, in fact, been fundamentally altered.

Outside the curtains we use to hide the dead, nothing has changed. The normalcy of the outside world feels somehow suspicious. Mundane scenes like a housekeeper mopping or a group of people laughing immediately feel awkward or even inappropriate given the immediate context. It was within this landscape that I continued to see my new patients.

The next patient had been waiting a long time. Triaged

before the dead woman had even arrived, she was upset about the delay in her care.

I introduced myself.

"Hello." I smiled for her benefit. "My name is Dr. Nahvi. This is Daniela. We work with your nurse, Isabel, who you've already met. We're part of the team that's going to take care of you. So tell me, what brings you in today?"

She immediately scolded me.

"Finally! I've been waiting *forever*," she moaned. "What in the world is going on here? Why did it take so long for you to come?"

Before medical school, I spent years working in restaurants as a waiter and bartender. I worked those jobs simply to support myself, yet the skills I picked up along the way proved to be surprisingly useful in the emergency room. My medical school classes may have taught me the particulars of human anatomy and physiology, but they never addressed how one might go about converting a stranger's impatient frustration into a calm understanding. The truth is, I often go weeks in the emergency room without calling upon a single lesson taught in my embryology or genetics classes, but an hour never passes where I do not employ the skills I have honed as a waiter.

On this day, however, I could not bring myself to apply those skills. The previous patient's death still loomed unsettled in my heart and mind, and I became reflexively irritated. The complaint felt insensitive given the context of my experience. "Count your blessings," I wanted to tell her. "In the bigger picture, your problem is not so bad."

Of course, this reaction was unfair. This particular patient was completely unaware that another patient had died. She did not know that the husband was grieving and that some of the hospital's staff were now silently running through their own emotions. Indeed, we had hidden all this from her in order that she not know. All of our patients in the emergency room are already ill or otherwise anxious, so we purposefully try our best not to remind them that death is indeed a possible outcome of an emergency room visit. We hide our dead bodies. We smile bravely and develop euphemisms. We substitute coded messages on our overhead announcements like, "Code blue in room fourteen, please. Code blue in room fourteen, please."

The code system allows the hospital to announce critical issues over their public address systems for employees to hear, while shielding patients and visitors from whatever grim news these codes may represent. "Code Blue," for example, might signify that somewhere in the hospital a patient has lost their pulse or their ability to breathe, while "Code Black" might indicate that a mass casualty incident has taken place.

Over time, however, this lexicon of codes has become so thoroughly absorbed into hospital culture that the word "code" alone has become synonymous with death itself. And so, in the local dialect of the emergency room, a patient who has died is simply said to have "coded," while a physician who is busy attempting the resuscitation of a dead patient is said to be off "running a code." In this way, what was once a metaphor has swallowed up and become what it formerly merely represented.

"Sorry, we had an emergency and we've been a little backed up tonight," I offered in my defense.

The woman rolled her eyes at me. "Isn't everything in the emergency room an emergency?"

It was a technicality, but she had a point.

I asked again about her symptoms.

She told me how for the past three days she had had a runny nose, that it got worse when she lay down flat and better when she sat upright. She told me that she had an itchy throat and a dry cough, and felt generally crummy, but that she did not have a fever and was still able to eat and drink and breathe and walk normally. She told me that she had not traveled outside the country recently. She denied feeling any chest pain or any abdominal pain. She told me that she had not passed out, nor did she suffer from any other medical conditions. She told me that she hadn't yet tried any medications to alleviate her symptoms. She told me that her five-year-old son and her seven-year-old daughter were recently ill with the same symptoms she now had.

In short, she told me that she had a common cold.

I smiled wearily, told her that she was going to be okay, and prescribed her some over-the-counter ibuprofen. I advised her to follow up with her primary care doctor and to come back if anything changed.

She seemed unsatisfied. I shrugged and walked off.

I made a mental note to score a point for the puppy dog team. When Cute Puppy bests Medical Degree, it is sometimes because we have simply forfeited the game.

Oscillating between mortality and minor illness is a staple of our work, yet it is a feeling I have never become accustomed to. It is hard to know what to make of a patient with a runny nose when only seconds earlier another patient just took her last breath. Put very bluntly, it is hard to care.

I understood that this patient only wanted to feel better. I understood that she probably knew I could not cure her cold and that she only wanted to tell her story and to be heard. I understood that she was as deserving of understanding, compassion, and care as any other patient. And yet I also understood that whatever I did, she would soon be completely well while my dead patient would remain dead. The emotional disconnect of such a circumstance is tremendous. It is difficult to muster the appropriate concern for one patient's mild discomforts after one has already spent so much emotional reserve helping a dead patient's husband navigate an existential crisis.

I knew that I should care, but I could not bring myself to. In situations like these, one cannot help but view the present moment through the lens of the immediate past. It is moments like these, I came to appreciate over the years, that are the real challenge of work in the emergency room. It is not dealing with the blood of a gunshot wound or the jagged bones of a trauma victim. It is not working the weekend and overnight shifts or the vast amounts of information that must be internalized and called upon on a moment's notice. Nor is it the mere stress of death, no matter how often I am asked how I deal with it. What ultimately makes life in the emergency room challenging is the extent to which we experience big and profound events, and lack the ability to process them. Over and over, we are deeply embedded in scenarios that have no answer. They leave us feeling tired, conflicted and confused.

We know that death must occur and that, by virtue of our

work, we must be a part of it. We know that our patients will have common colds and that we must be a part of those experiences as well. But, somehow, these elements, when combined, seem to make no sense at all.

We can appreciate each tree for precisely what it is, yet no matter how we squint our eyes, the forest seems to remain blurry.

NINE

EVEN OUR PRINCIPLES STUMBLE

The emergency room is full of strange and perplexing scenarios. At every turn, we see principles that we have long held become challenged. We see problems that have no solution and conflicts for which there exist no good outcome. We see that there are, in fact, many things in our world that are unclear and uncomfortable and for which we have no answers. We are unsure what to make of them.

It is not that what we see in the emergency room is unique. Quite the opposite: the emergency room is the front porch of society. As is baked into our ethos and backed by federal law,[1] any person is welcome at our door at any time to have any problem addressed. As such, the emergency room is simply all of us.

What makes the emergency room special is that it takes our common problems—the same people and circumstances that we see in our everyday lives—and presents them after they have been ratcheted up to their furthest extremes. This is due to the simple fact that while the emergency room is open to everyone, nobody actually wants to be in one. The emergency room is a place of last resort. One ends up in an emergency room only when every other better option has failed—when a medical problem is too severe for a doctor's office or when a homeless man shivering in the winter cold is turned away from every shelter, with nowhere to go.

At an emergency room that I previously worked in, there was a patient who arrived annually on the Fourth of July. Every year, he refused medical care and brushed aside any suggestion that he speak with a psychiatrist. In fact, he dismissed any efforts we offered him that would have allowed us to intervene in any way. Instead, his only request was to be allowed to stay in a patient room for the duration of the day. He respectfully requested a room farthest away from any windows or doors, but made sure to state that he would be grateful for any room that we were able to offer him. Having grown up in the nearby housing projects, where he saw many of his friends and neighbors fall victim to gun violence, his only request was that we allow him to wait out the day in peace in some safe corner of the emergency room until the cacophony of the fireworks outside had abated.

For three hundred and sixty-four days of the year, this patient is our ordinary neighbor, coworker, or someone we may pass on the street. On this lone day every year, however, with nowhere else to go, the emergency department becomes his refuge. He has no interest in what we have to offer—indeed, he does not wish to be in the emergency room at all—and yet, in order to escape whatever it is he needs escaping from among the loud bangs and crackles every Independence Day, he finds himself returning year after year.

In this way, we routinely see patients only after they have exhausted every other avenue society has given them and when they do not know where else to turn. It is not that we see unique problems in the emergency room, but rather, that we see common problems uniquely presented.

In simple terms, the emergency room is more. It is the same song we hear on a daily basis, only louder. And just as we may nod our heads and tap our feet to a song that is quietly playing in the background only to find it completely off-putting when it is cranked up to its highest volume, the same is true for so many things in our day-to-day lives. When life's volume is turned up to its highest level, what was previously firm and stable can suddenly become shaky and uncertain. The same dilemmas we may have previously made little note of suddenly become difficult to ignore. We may find that the basic assumptions we have long relied on to guide our decisions are more nuanced than we appreciated. We may find that, at their extremes, the fundamental principles upon which we build our entire lives are not so straightforward.

For example, we may think that it is obvious when we would stop a resuscitation attempt and pronounce a person dead, that if the brain cannot survive more than thirty minutes without oxygen then, of course, we would stop our efforts at that point. But when we are in the middle of a resuscitation attempt, faced not just with death but also with the collateral damage it leaves in its wake, we find that, somehow, what we ning.

know does not translate to what we actually do. We may find that it is possible to pursue either of two utterly dichotomous courses of action and that both of them may be correct.

I recall one of the first times I came to appreciate how unsteady our life's principles are when I was a resident in training. I was rotating through my hospital's internal medicine wards, caring for a patient who was particularly suited to test my very notion of right and wrong.

This patient had a high-end handbag by her bedside, but it was filled with nothing but crumpled receipts and loose cigarettes. Her hair was disheveled, as if it had not been brushed in days. Her skin was slightly yellowed, and her abdomen was protuberant. She smelled of vomit and was curled up into a ball in her hospital bed, quietly snoring.

I remember checking the name on her wristband so that I could address her.

"Ms. Riley?"

No response.

"Ms. Riley!" I tried again.

This time she seemed to stir. Without opening her eyes, she moved her head, offered several incomprehensible mumbles, and went back to sleep.

"MS. RILEY!!" I said, putting a hand on her sternum, now shaking her.

"WHAT?! Why are you shouting?!"

I began to speak with her but stopped again when I realized she was sleeping once more.

In order to communicate with her, I would have to continuously rock her entire body while we spoke. The moment

I let go, she would go to sleep. She was like a two-way radio that would shut off the instant the "talk" button was released. To engage in dialogue, I would have to constantly press down.

"Ms. Riley," I said, fine-tuning my continuous jostles and disturbing her just enough to prevent her from going to sleep. "How do you feel today?"

"I'm fine, leave me alone," she mumbled, swatting my hand off her chest.

Unable to obtain anything of substance from her, I went to our electronic medical record for help. I learned from her medical history that Ms. Riley was not simply drunk or tired. Ms. Riley was sleepy and confused as a result of her medical condition. I learned that she used to be a lawyer in Connecticut. She had been a functional alcoholic, until one day she no longer was.

Now simply an alcoholic without the benefit of a modifying adjective, Ms. Riley was unable to work or keep an apartment. She had no family, and no healthcare proxy. From her drinking, Ms. Riley had caused permanent damage to her liver, resulting in frequent admissions to the hospital for a disease known as hepatic encephalopathy. In short, her liver was no longer able to clean up the natural toxins that flowed through her bloodstream; as they accumulated, those toxins would go to her brain, making her confused, sleepy, and unable to care for herself. Left untreated, she could eventually slip into a coma and die.

Luckily, the treatment for hepatic encephalopathy is very effective. Unluckily, however, it is yet another example of modern medicine's terrible trade-offs—a miracle with an asterisk and plenty of fine print. One of the main medications we use, lactulose, is simultaneously highly effective and highly undesirable. Lactulose works by creating explosive diarrhea.

That unfortunate response is not a side effect. Explosive diarrhea is precisely how lactulose is designed to function. Mimicking the effect that lactose has on individuals who are lactose intolerant, lactulose cannot be broken down and digested. The indigestible molecules cause those who ingest it to experience bloating, flatulence, and diarrhea, which, in turn, serves to eliminate toxins like ammonia before the body has the chance to absorb them. In a sense, it is a detox cleanse.

Like a mad scientist ignoring the means he employs to reach his desired end, the appropriate dose of lactulose is calculated not by a set number of ounces or milligrams, but by a set number of bowel movements. The *goal* is to reach three loose bowel movements per day. Too much diarrhea and we decrease the dose—too little and we increase it. What this ultimately means is that for this lifesaving medication to work, the patient necessarily exists in a perpetual state of discomfort. Most patients who are prescribed lactulose hate to take it, despite understanding that it has the potential to save their life.

"Ms. Riley, you need to take your lactulose," I told her. "Your encephalopathy is getting worse and it's starting to get dangerous. You can barely stay awake."

"No! I don't want it! Shut up and leave me alone."

"Ms. Riley, do you know where we are? Do you know what kind of place this is? Do you know who I am?" I asked, testing her with a pop quiz that should have been insultingly easy. I was wearing a white coat with a name tag, had a stethoscope around my neck, and was flanked by IV poles, EKG machines, and oxygen tanks. These were hardly trick questions.

Nevertheless, she was unable to answer any of them. She had no clue where—or even when—we were.

"Ms. Riley, it's no problem if you don't want to take it, but can you at least tell me *why* we want you to take your lactulose? Can you tell us what could happen if you don't take it?"

Once again, she had no answer.

When it became clear that she could not pass our most basic of tests, Ms. Riley crossed an invisible ethical line that changed her hospital trajectory. Demonstrating that she was too confused to know where she was, what was going on around her, or even the basic consequences of her decisions, Ms. Riley had given up her autonomy. She was so confused that ethically—and legally as well—she could no longer be her own caretaker. From here on, her words would be considered, but we would be making decisions on her behalf.

In medical parlance, the principle on which this hinges is known as "decision-making capacity." When a patient is deemed to have it, they can make decisions as they like, even as we vehemently disagree with them. When they do not have it, however, they are stripped of this authority.

In the emergency room, this principle is most commonly invoked in the setting of alcohol use. It is not uncommon, for example, for drunk patients to violently resist our help when they arrive. They may be suffering from traumatic injuries— the shattered ankles and brain bleeds that alcohol intoxication so often seems to play a role in—and yet, in their stupor, they may refuse our efforts to help. Often, their reasons seem silly. They may complain that they do not want our help because they do not want us to cut away their favorite article of clothing with our shears. "Stop! Leave me alone! No way! That's my favorite jacket!" they might protest as we cut it off so we can assess them for a stab wound. Alternatively, their reasons might be dismissive. They may simply swat us away, asking to be left alone so they can rest. "I'm fine, go away. I just want to sleep," they might mumble as blood soaks through their hair and into their hospital bedsheets.

Often, however, after their bleeding arteries have been tied and their injuries have been addressed—long after they have sobered up—these patients apologize for their behavior and thank us for ignoring their objections.

Knowing that this is often how things play out, we do not listen to people who are unable to understand what they are saying. It is not worth the risk of having them die over a nap or a leather coat. In this way, many lives have been saved over the protests of those who needed saving.

It should be made clear, however, that a person who *does* retain decision-making capacity is permitted to make any decision they like. We have no interest in forcibly treating someone who has no interest in what it is we have to offer. Furthermore, it is remarkably easy for one to demonstrate that they retain capacity. Patients need not exhibit any sort of sophistication or deep medical literacy, but merely the most basic understanding of whatever decision they are making. If, for example, in the midst of a heart attack, a patient who did not wish to obtain treatment for his heart attack were able to tell us that forgoing treatment could lead to a progressive and worsening heart attack, he would be determined to retain decision-making capacity. It is, admittedly, a low bar. Upon surmounting it, one is free to make whatever decision they wish. Ultimately, it is a simple standard that any smart five-year-old should be able to pass.[2]

While it might feel troubling to allow such a patient to walk out the door injured and untreated, it is the right thing to do. The alternative—holding someone who simply disagrees with our conclusions against their will and treating them against their refusals—would be far worse. Such an action would, effectively, be imprisonment.

Despite these complexities, the idea of decision-making capacity is nothing more than a codified default-to-life. When someone cannot demonstrate that they recognize the gravity of their own situation, we *assume* that they want to stay alive, whatever they may do or say.

Because Ms. Riley failed this most basic test, she would be getting her lactulose.

By the next day, Ms. Riley's mental state improved. The medicines were beginning to work. She became alert and oriented and was able to hold normal conversation. As a result, Ms. Riley regained her decision-making capacity. She had become her own boss once more.

Remarkably, however, her newfound alertness did not affect her ultimate calculations. When it was offered to her, Ms. Riley continued to refuse her lactulose.

She told the team caring for her that it was not that she

wanted to die, but that, very simply, she did not want to live with the constant discomfort that her lactulose necessitated. She told us that she understood the consequences, but that she simply hated feeling bloated all day, every day. Whatever we may have thought of her decision, it was clear that this was the considered conclusion that she had come to.

Now, however, despite her answer being unchanged from the previous day, we could no longer administer Ms. Riley's medications over her objections. And so, after improving during her hospital stay, Ms. Riley would be discharged without the medications she needed.

Inevitably, after leaving without her medications, Ms. Riley decompensated once more. She became ill once again. She ended up back in the emergency room. And we repeated the same sequence of events as before.

Over the next few months, Ms. Riley repeatedly found herself in the same place and in the same state. Each time, our hospital would provide her with lifesaving medications despite her refusals, and each time, she would improve until she was able to refuse medication. She would leave, worsen, and return. We would repeat the process until it became a sort of charade.

It was, however, not unreasonable. Ms. Riley's decision to refuse her medications was not entirely irrational. While I may have come to a different conclusion than she did, I understood why she came to hers.

Amazingly, the ethical principles and laws that got us into such a mess were not broken, wrong, or bad. It was simply that, with the tools available to us, Ms. Riley's problem existed beyond our ability to address them in any rational way. She somehow lived in a state beyond the reach of any rational approach. Ms. Riley existed outside of logic itself.

Should we have forced her to take her medications when she was deemed able to refuse, we would have become authoritarians. Should we have held them from her when she was deemed unfit to understand her situation simply because we knew she had refused her medications in the past, we would have become cruel samaritans, giving up on a human life and on the hope that a person could change their mind and their ways. And so, by way of doing everything right, Ms. Riley's life nevertheless became an inescapable Sisyphean feedback loop. By everything working as it should, everything somehow still went wrong.

This was one of the first times in medicine that I walked away truly unsure of how to feel. Proud of our dedication to her potential to improve, I was nevertheless frustrated that we were putting so much energy into something that seemed so futile. Content to apply our best principles to navigate our difficult path, I was disappointed to find how weak and feeble those principles seemed to be when taken to their furthest extreme.

I would quickly learn, however, that such circumstances—situations where nothing actually goes wrong and yet, at the same time, nothing goes quite right—are not uncommon. Through the nature of our work, we encounter them almost routinely.

I recall caring for a patient named Ms. Hill. She was brought to us by ambulance after having passed out and fallen to the ground at her nursing home.

Despite her fall, Ms. Hill claimed that she was without pain or injury. She told me that she felt great and that she had no complaints at all. She told me that she could not actually remember having fallen to begin with. She told me, in fact, that she could not remember very much of anything at all.

Well into her eighties, Ms. Hill was suffering from a good degree of dementia. She had identified the hospital as an "arena" and believed we were living in the era of the Sputnik launches. She was absentminded and would reply to our questions with upbeat but irrelevant answers that were often untethered to reality.

"How are you feeling today?" was asked.

"I'm feeling great! As long as I take my pills I'm doing wonderfully," Ms. Hill replied, appearing to make perfect sense at first.

"That sounds fantastic—did you take your pills today?"

"Of course I do. I take them every day."

"And just so I know which pills we're talking about, could you tell me which medications you take, just to make sure everything we have in our computer is up-to-date?"

"Oh, I don't know, I just take whichever ones that Jerry gives me."

An aide from the nursing home who had accompanied her looked toward me to obtain eye contact and quietly shook her head no, as if to say, "Don't believe this."

I picked up on the cue. "That's terrific. Who is Jerry?"

Soon she was giving us a detailed and loving description of her dead husband, who she believed was somehow still caring for her and administering her medications. Ms. Hill did not know which pills she took, was not sure where they came from, what they were intended to treat, or how she obtained them at all. She did not even seem to realize that she was living in a nursing home.

Nevertheless, despite her dementia, Ms. Hill was exceedingly merry. As long as we did not venture into any details or specifics, we were able to engage in delightful conversation. She demonstrated as much concern for me as I did for her, and she dispensed sweet compliments to the nurses and technicians like candy on Halloween. When I asked if there was anything that might be hurting or bothering her, she laughed me off and merely responded by saying how fantastic she felt. On a scale of bad to good, Ms. Hill considered everything some degree of "super."

If one considers the ultimate goal of life to be a happy and contented existence, Ms. Hill seemed to have taken a shortcut. Without having to attend to the circumstances of her life, she had somehow arrived at the goal. She existed, it seemed, happily.

Nevertheless, tasked with caring for Ms. Hill's well-being and refusing to put much stock in her self-assessment that she was "completely fine," we conducted a thorough evaluation. We checked her body for injuries that may have resulted from her fall, and we drew blood tests to assess for any anomalies that might have led to it. Upon plugging Ms. Hill in to our cardiac monitoring machines, we identified her problem.

Ms. Hill's heart was beating in a dangerous and unstable

rhythm. Known as ventricular tachycardia, it was the type of rhythm that not only was the likely cause of her collapse in her nursing home, but also had the potential to lead to her sudden death. And so, while Ms. Hill would speak, laugh, and tell stories, she might have perished at any moment. Having found the source of our problem, we hurried along to attach her to tubes that would deliver boluses of medications and machines that could deliver loads of electricity to address it. As we did this, however, a nurse brought a piece of paperwork to our attention.

It was her advance directives. Ms. Hill had a "Do Not Resuscitate" order in place as well as a set of specific instructions for what we should—and should not—do in the event of an emergency like the one we found ourselves in today.

Advance directives are documents that patients generate when they are well, in order to instruct healthcare providers what to do on their behalf when they are not. As it is our default to take aggressive action, these documents are generally designed not to tell us what to do for our patients, but what *not* to do.

Often, patients may ask us not to intervene on their behalf after they have been diagnosed with incurable diseases such as end-stage cancer or a progressive dementia like the one Ms. Hill was diagnosed with. These patients understand that even if our interventions stave off death today, they will do nothing to change the outlook for tomorrow. These patients often tell us that rather than continuing to live in a state of pain or debility—knowing that each subsequent day will bring more troubles than the last—they would prefer to be allowed to "die a natural death."

Regardless of their specific reasons, patients who file advance directives have taken a hard look at what modern medicine has to offer, have considered its merits, and have decided to reject the offer. It is often our most well-informed patients who want the least done on their behalf.

Glancing over the paperwork that was handed to me as we rushed to fix her condition, I noted that Ms. Hill's advance directives specifically included a clause that precluded us from treating her in this moment. Should her heart find itself in an unstable rhythm, her paperwork had instructed, we were not to correct it. Effectively, Ms. Hill had anticipated the exact scenario she found herself in, and had requested that we not intervene. What this practically meant, of course, is that whatever happened over the next few moments, we could do nothing but watch. It was possible that we would be carrying on pleasant, if untethered, conversation with Ms. Hill right until the moment she died.

I called Ms. Hill's daughter on the phone.

I informed her of her mother's situation. I asked if she would come to the emergency room in order to be with her, and I requested that she confirm that the paperwork her mother had in place was accurate.

She sighed. "My mother's had a tough time these past few months," she said. "We knew this day would come sooner or later."

She calmly confirmed that the documents were accurate and that, as her mother's healthcare proxy, she agreed with them. She told us she was on her way to the hospital to be with her mother.

Finally, I went over to speak to Ms. Hill herself. My previous interactions suggested that the conversation would be a strange one. I would be informing a woman who believed we were currently living about a half century in the past that she was critically ill and might soon die. I would inform her that she herself had previously asked that we not intervene on her behalf, and I would try to confirm whether that request was still accurate. I was not quite sure what to expect.

"Ms. Hill," I began, "I have a bit of news for you."

"Oh?" She smiled inquisitively.

"It looks like the reason you passed out and fell at your nursing home is because your heart is in quite an unstable rhythm. It's something called ventricular tachycardia—to be honest, it's pretty dangerous."

"Oh." She raised her eyebrows, giving off the slightest hint of alarm.

"I'm worried that your heart might not be able to keep this up for too long and, eventually—maybe even soon—it might stop. Of course, that would be deadly."

"Oh my." She repeated herself twice.

"Now, I looked through your records and I spoke with your daughter and noticed that you have a set of advance directives and a Do Not Resuscitate order in place. It seems like the treatments that we would normally give you for this are treatments that you have decided you would not want."

Upon speaking these words, I immediately became anxious. Having already verified my obligations with Ms. Hill's daughter, I wondered what I would do if Ms. Hill herself now disagreed? I worried that, in the course of our discussion,

Ms. Hill might express some vague disagreement with what was outlined in her paperwork and what was confirmed by her daughter, which would muddle my obligations. In such a case, I wondered, would it be better to respect the wishes she herself had previously expressed when she was in a sound state of mind—indeed, the wishes she had specifically expressed upon anticipating this exact scenario—or would it be better to respect the wishes that she expressed now, despite, perhaps, not fully understanding them? How coherent does one have to be, after all, to determine that they want to continue to live?

My anxieties were spared.

"Oh. Yes, that's right, I don't want any of that. Whatever my daughter says is correct; you can just listen to her."

And so, somehow, I found myself breathing a sigh of relief upon hearing an elderly lady give permission for the possibility of her imminent death.

As much as my dilemma with Ms. Hill centered on her acceptance of death, there are patients who trouble us for precisely the opposite reason. I will never forget the haunting experience I had while caring for an elderly patient named Ms. Price when I was in medical school.

Like Ms. Hill, Ms. Price was suffering from dementia. Unlike Ms. Hill, however, Ms. Price's dementia had progressed far beyond her being simply confused and disoriented.

Long past the point where she could recognize the correct time or place, Ms. Price had lost her ability to recognize anything at all. Often, as we walked into the room, she would not look at us, but instead, stare slack-jawed straight through us. She failed to recognize our presence. Ms. Price had lost many of her functional capacities. She had been admitted to the hospital, in fact, after she had begun to lose her very instincts to eat and drink. Her dementia had so thoroughly ravaged her brain that she no longer registered the sensations of hunger or thirst.

Even worse, in addition to forgetting to eat and drink, Ms. Price was also forgetting *how* to perform these actions. The smooth muscles in her esophagus had begun to fail her, and what she swallowed in her mouth was no longer guaranteed to end up in her stomach. Ms. Price's dementia had progressed to the point that she had lost the very reflexes she had been born with. Now, during attempts to feed her, it was not uncommon for the food she swallowed to end up not in her gastrointestinal tract, where it belonged, but in her lungs, where it did not. Over the past several months, Ms. Price had suffered through several life-threatening episodes of pneumonia as a result.

Unlike Ms. Hill, Ms. Price had generated no advance directive and filed no Do Not Resuscitate order. She had not assigned any particular person as her healthcare proxy. And so, by the legal hierarchy enumerated by New York State's next-of-kin laws, her children were designated to make decisions on her behalf. Deeply devout in their faith, her children had decided not to make decisions for their mother alone, but in counsel with their religious leader. Upon doing so, they were informed that "all life is inherently valuable"—that no matter the state of existence that was being led, it was essential that everything be done to preserve a human life for as long as possible. And so, on their mother's behalf, they insisted on all efforts to keep her alive.

Tremendous efforts are undertaken to sustain the lives of patients like Ms. Price. After all, if eating itself has become a danger, one must find a way to administer food while bypassing the very act of swallowing. This requires the surgical insertion of a gastric tube.

Ms. Price was admitted to the hospital for the procedure. Going forward, rather than having to remember to eat, she would be provided with food intermittently throughout the day. Her food would arrive as a thick liquid in a clear plastic bottle, which an aide would insert directly into the plastic port by her abdomen that served as a conduit to her stomach. On rare occasions, as a sort of treat our medical system refers to as "leisure feeds," an aide would occasionally slather her lips and tongue with a spoon covered with minute amounts of food so that Ms. Price could enjoy the bliss of taste.

Patients like this are not uncommon in the large academic hospitals of New York City. What made this particular patient so memorable, however, was the chilling soundtrack that occasionally played in her hospital room.

Mostly nonverbal and certainly unable to hold a conversation, Ms. Price still retained the ability to speak single words and short phrases. Often they appeared nonsensical and out of context. Nevertheless, every once in a while, Ms. Price would stare straight ahead and repeat the phrase "kill me" in a frail and raspy voice. With or without an audience, through thick white dregs caking the corners of her mouth, staring straight ahead and directing her words to nobody in particular, she would intermittently repeat the phrase. I remember, as a medical student, standing in the hallway outside her room while conducting our morning rounds only to hear her repeat the phrase, "kill me, kill me," in a slow monotone in her empty hospital room.

"I know, it's super creepy, but just ignore her," I remember the resident physician who was then my supervisor telling me. "She doesn't know what she's saying and her children are making decisions on her behalf and they are insistent that 'everything be done.'"

It was impossible, of course, to guess the extent to which Ms. Price understood the words she was saying, let alone how much she could have meant them. There was no way of knowing whether Ms. Price was truly suicidal, or, perhaps, speaking the phrase arbitrarily, no different than if she were to randomly utter "cookie dough" or "blue balloon." Furthermore, no matter what we may have thought of her statement and her condition, it was not we but her children—those who loved her and knew her best and who were guided by their shared faith and value system—who would make the most appropriate decisions on her behalf. Thus we did exactly as my supervising resident directed. We ignored her raspy pleas.

We continued our therapies. We poked and prodded her, we drew her blood and urine, and our surgeons performed whatever procedures might have been needed in order to keep her organs functioning. We applied whatever technologies we had to maintain her physical survival.

Like Ms. Hill's before her, Ms. Price's story raises questions. Both situations, of course, were discomfiting. Yet both of them stirred me for opposing reasons. While the circumstance of one patient troubled me because of her acceptance of death, the circumstance of another was troubling because of her family's refusal to consider it.

It is deceptively easy while in the process of caring for either of these patients to think, *This feels wrong*. It is much harder, however, to come up with a better course of action. To preserve life would necessarily come at the cost of creating more suffering. And in order to minimize suffering we would have to give up on the idea of preserving life. At best, we could only honor one principle at the expense of another. Ms. Hill and Ms. Price were effectively the same patient, only at different stages in their disease.

Ultimately, their example confirms what we already know: life sometimes contains no perfect solutions and no "correct" courses of action. We are often surrounded by unknowns, and yet, we must take action. We are routinely presented with the impossible situation where there exists no right thing to do.

Importantly, none of the challenges and ideas in this chapter are unique to the emergency room. They are the same principles that guide us in our day-to-day lives. The ideas that life should be preserved, that individuals should be able to make decisions on their own behalf, that human suffering should be alleviated, that we should hold out hope that people can change for the better, and that we should be respectful of the decisions that others make even when we disagree are basic, fundamental beliefs that we all hold. But these beliefs look somewhat different when life's volume has been turned up.

In this way, I have come to learn, that as much as our code blues and code blacks may capture our attention, it is ultimately the code grays that we experience—the subtle moments where what we feel and believe about the world itself is put to the test—that are the most important dramas we face in the emergency room and beyond.

TEN

A DECIDEDLY UNORTHODOX CHAPTER

I realize, dear reader, that throughout the course of this book I have raised a series of issues for which no solutions exist. I do not want to create the impression that those issues will be addressed and epiphanies will emerge. They will not. There will be no grand resolution to the issues I have raised.

I also realize that many of the stories I have recounted are not necessarily uplifting. Depicting strange and sometimes troubling dilemmas does not make for particularly airy reading. You might ask, then, what is the point of telling these stories?

Frankly, it is to make us uncomfortable.

Too often in life we come across issues that could present us with a moment of appreciation, reflection, or growth. But too often we simply move on—to the next patient, the next task, the next day of work—noting the magnitude of the issue before us, but failing to internalize it in any meaningful way. Too often we scroll through our smartphones for the duration of a forty-five-second elevator ride, preferring the dopamine of our mindlessness over the discomforts of our unresolved thoughts.

I believe it is worth seeing our strange and uncomfortable experiences for what they are. It is only through acknowledging our discomforts that we can sort through our thoughts and understand our world in a more meaningful way. It is only through acknowledging our discomforts that we can reflect on our lives and consider what it is that is truly important within them. And it is only through acknowledging our discomforts that we can reject the notion that the way things are is the way they ought to be.

These stories, then, allow us to play in the sandbox of our discomfort. They allow us to pause to examine the strange quirks and impossible challenges and subtle beauties of life. They allow us to better appreciate life itself, and they force us to question things we may have previously taken for granted. They allow us to consider the rawness of our human experience and are a reminder that we might be better off if we focused less on our day-to-day distractions and more on the things that are truly meaningful to us.

So at the end of the day, I do not believe the appropriate question is "what is the point" of these stories, but precisely the opposite: What is the point of going through life without exploring stories such as these? What is the point of leading an unexamined life?

With all this in mind, I leave you not with any details or any answers, but with this decidedly unorthodox chapter. As you read these stories I ask that you consider that perhaps there is something to gain from becoming more comfortable with our discomforts.

PART II

But Reason was a useless judge,
And answers? He had none.

—Hafez, *Faces of Love*, trans. Dick Davis

ELEVEN

THE COUGH THAT WAS CANCER

Back in the emergency room, my dead patient's husband finally walked over and pulled me aside.

"Okay, I'm ready to talk now if you're free."

I asked Daniela to take him to a private room while I went to collect supplies for our conversation. I turned off my phone and traded my stethoscope and penlight for a jug of ice water and a box of tissues. Working in the hospital as a medical scribe, Daniela was also a premedical student. I invited her in to observe the conversation.

"It's certainly not fun," I warned. "But if you're interested in doing this for the rest of your life, it's probably good to see all the different parts of the job."

Glad to be involved, she eagerly agreed.

I thought of the first time I had to navigate a difficult conversation with a patient.

This particular patient was in her forties, and had come to

the ER to be evaluated for a chronic cough. She had already gone to her primary care doctor, who, appropriately, had obtained an x-ray. It was read as normal. She was nevertheless prescribed a course of antibiotics to see if they would help her improve. They did not.

As her cough persisted, she presented to the emergency room requesting further evaluation. This patient had none of the secondary signs that would suggest a more insidious problem that a persistent cough might signify—she suffered no weight loss, no night sweats, no chills, for example—but we decided to pursue a CT scan anyway. As Danny, the physician assistant, might have said, "something just didn't feel right."

I placed a series of orders and went on to evaluate other patients who were waiting. Soon her results began to trickle back. The results of her blood tests came back as normal, and her vital signs revealed a blood pressure that was better than my own. Before the result of the CT scan became available on our electronic medical record, however, I heard an overhead announcement.

"Radiology on line three for Dr. Nahvi. Radiology on line three."

Radiologists work alone and in dimmed rooms. Their job is very different from our work in the emergency room. They spend hours reviewing pictures of bones, brains, and bowels. They spend their days seeing *representations* of patients, but rarely see those patients themselves. Radiologists rarely even get to see other doctors. When a radiologist makes the effort for a live conversation, one can be certain that something is amiss. Radiologists rarely call just to say hello.

I picked up the phone.

"Hey, Alice Carter from radiology here. Are you the doctor taking care of patient Wallace?" the radiologist began.

I was.

"Great, well, there's no pneumonia or pulmonary embolism, if that's what you were looking for . . ."

I was not, I thought to myself as it became clear that another shoe was about to drop.

". . . but she does have a bunch of ground-glass opacities and some big nodules all over the place. And it's pretty limited since we didn't scan all the way down to the abdomen, but from what I can see of the liver in this study, it looks like she has a couple of spots there as well . . ."

Despite the ambiguity of her language thus far, it became clear what this portended.

"I can't tell what the primary is from the CT scan, but it looks like it's probably lung," she continued. "Either way—wherever it's coming from—she has metastatic cancer. It's all over the place. Sad. What a bummer, no? Looks like she's pretty young. Anyway, before we go, can you spell your last name for me? I just need to document that we had this conversation. Thanks so much."

I was an intern at the time, just beginning my career. I understood that my next task was to walk over and tell the patient what we had found. I had, of course, anticipated that telling patients the news of a CT scan's unwelcome results would be part of my job. Until that point, however, I had never had to do such a thing. Somehow, I had believed that when the time came, I would be ready.

I was not.

I hung up the phone. I told my supervising resident what the radiologist had informed me and mentioned that I would be walking over to deliver the news of a cancer diagnosis to our young patient. He asked me if I had ever done such a thing before. I replied that I had not. Noting my inexperience, he asked me whether I felt comfortable having the conversation alone, or whether I might prefer that he join me. Projecting a sense of assuredness, I brushed him aside.

"No, no, I should be okay. Thanks, though."

My supervising resident gave me a thumbs-up. I interpreted it as his having confidence in my ability to go it alone, although, in hindsight, it is more likely that his reaction was simply one of relief at not having to become involved himself. Such encounters are never pleasant and one comes to appreciate the opportunity to avoid them if possible.

I went over the conversation in my head and was content with the strategy I had come up with. In my imagined conversation, I did a fantastic job. So, believing myself to be ready, I decided it was time to go over and tell this young woman that her cough was cancer.

My palms were sweaty. I walked over to a dispenser for some hand sanitizer to rub into my hands. It was a trick that I appreciated during the early months of my training. Hand sanitizer is ubiquitously available in the emergency room— with the press of a lever, an outward sign of anxiety can easily be concealed as a commitment to hand hygiene.

When I finally arrived at my patient's room, I asked her how she was doing. She flashed an anxious smile. My mind went blank. I stuttered and stumbled. I rambled for what felt like an eternity. I felt the need to couch each word that had a hint of a negativity with five others that were uplifting. I found myself unable to deny her the reassurance she had come in seeking. What terrified me most, I realized, was my fear of making her upset. Seeing her smile, I could not bring myself to say words that I knew would undo it.

Never before did I appreciate how powerful our instinct to console is. Understanding that she was anxious and was seeking reassurance, I desperately wanted to tell her that she was all right. Knowing that the news I had would be devastating, I did not want to deliver it.

In our day-to-day lives, we are used to providing reassurance. When friends or loved ones are anxious, it is second nature to tell them that things will work out and that everything will be okay. When things are bad, we tell them that things will get better. This is partially because it is what we want for them, but it is also because it is almost always true. Profound and permanent problems are, thankfully, rare. As a result, however, when we need to do it, we find it astoundingly difficult to actually confirm someone's deepest anxieties. We find ourselves fighting an instinct to tell them that everything will be okay.

As I wrapped up my conversation and began walking back to my computer terminal, I appreciated that my patient was still smiling. Reviewing everything in my mind, I realized that my desire to avoid letting her down had become so profound that I had completely failed my actual task. Somehow, I realized, I had navigated the entire conversation and avoided uttering the word "cancer" entirely.

Instead, I had told her that there "were findings" on the CT scan that "looked like masses."

She asked me what "those masses" could represent.

I told her that the masses could reflect "a lot of things" and that "some of those things" could be "very bad."

She had asked me what types of bad things the masses could represent. I retreated. I told her, "Well, they *could* be something really dangerous." But "it's hard to say."

"You're probably going to need a biopsy to definitively say for sure what they are," I told her.

Indeed, it was literally hard for me to say it. While it was technically true—her CT scan *would* have to be followed by a biopsy in order to prove that the masses were, in fact, cancer—the reality was that I was hedging in order to avoid my responsibility. In order to avoid making her upset, I clung to a hope that did not reasonably exist. Barring some bizarre and exceedingly unlikely alternate explanation, I knew that she had cancer.

I also knew that the real reason I hedged and deflected was in the hope that some other doctor would have to tell her that she had cancer. If I could convince myself that she did not have cancer until a biopsy proved it, then the responsibility of informing her of her diagnosis fell upon the doctor who would order her biopsy. I was, of course, passing the buck. Using desperate mental leaps, I had somehow justified to myself that this would be the right thing to do. Using the word "cancer," I told myself in the middle of that conversation, would be too overwhelming. *Better to simply plant the seed so that someone else could finish the conversation that I had begun*, I rationalized. I made several such excuses in an attempt to redefine my role and free myself from responsibility.

When I returned from my interaction and was sitting back down by my computer, my supervising resident asked me how the conversation went.

"It went okay," I lied. "But actually, I only started the conversation. I need to go back to finish it."

Aware that I had failed—and knowing that I would have to go back to do better—I knew that the conversation was not actually over. I stood back up. I stopped by the dispenser for some hand sanitizer once again. Two pumps.

I walked back to speak with the patient once more. I apologized and told her that I was worried that I did not convey the information as well as I should have and that there was more that I had to tell her.

I sat down beside her, took a deep breath, and looked her in the eye. I told her that I spoke with our radiologist and that it looked like the diagnosis was perhaps more certain than what I had originally been able to convey. I told her that the results would still have to be confirmed, but that we believed that she most likely had metastatic cancer. I told her that there would be a long road ahead. I told her that she likely had plenty of important questions that I did not have the answers to at this moment. I told her that the entirety of my information was based on the results of the CT scan, which showed that she had spots that looked like cancer and that that cancer had spread. What type of cancer, which particular treatments she would need, how far along the disease had progressed, or even the coarse outlines of her prognosis—these were all important questions that I was sure she had, but that I would be unable to answer that day. I told her that she would be seeing more doctors who, in time, would be able to provide her more answers in what was undoubtedly a highly anxious time. I told her that she had cancer, and that we would do what we could to help her along the way.

I have learned that, in the midst of such difficult conversations, there are specific words that make our job especially challenging. While there exist many devastating illnesses and prognoses, some words have taken on a special place in our collective psyche. "Cancer" is one of these words. Because of its outsized significance in our culture, it can make us particularly uncomfortable. Nevertheless, when discussing such sensitive topics, it is critical to use these sensitive words. Euphemisms—"concerning masses" and "passed away," for example—are tools we use to soften our blows. They are a disservice. When reality itself is a harsh blow, we have no right to temper it. We can be there for our patients, we can console them, but it is wrong to alter the reality they are facing.

Indeed, the medical literature teaches us that these euphemisms serve only as points of confusion.[1, 2] Often, unless we use the words that are so difficult to say, patients and family members fail to internalize the fullness of our statements. We may tell them they have a "worrisome mass" in their breast "that looks to be malignant," for example, only for them to respond with "well, thank God it's not cancer."

An emergency physician friend once told me about an experience he had with the family members of a patient who had died. He had pronounced the death of an elderly man and informed his family that their father had "passed away." He told me that they had a long conversation in which he delivered the news and that he then walked away to continue to treat other patients. This friend told me that several minutes later, his patient's family flagged him down once more and asked him to come over to speak with them. He asked what he could do to help.

"We talked it over and we want you to keep trying," this family told my friend.

"Trying what?" he asked them.

"We want you to continue trying to save him," they responded.

In their grief, this family failed to internalize the depth of the conversation that was just had. They failed to fully grasp that when he told them that their loved one had "passed away," it meant that he had died and that this death was final.

Ultimately, using anything but honest and frank language is not something that we do for our patients, but for ourselves. We may believe we are softening our blows for our audience but we know that, in the end, doing so does not actually help them. Like the old-fashioned doctors who used to take loved ones out of their dying family members' hospital rooms, we do this to avoid our own discomfort.

I asked my patient if she had any questions.

She asked about the results of the other tests we ran, referring to her blood and urine samples.

"Well, those tests are actually completely normal," I replied quickly, eager for the opportunity to deliver news of a normal test result.

"Oh great," she said. I remember her laughing at my answer.

Her reaction was understandable. When the engine of a car has cracked, it does little good to know that the air-conditioning is working just fine.

She told me that she never smoked, she ate a healthy diet, and that she exercised every day. She asked me why she would get lung cancer.

I did not have an answer.

She asked me if she was going to die.

I was caught off guard. "We all do," was the best reply I could come up with.

She cried and I sat by her bedside.

As Daniela and I were about to walk over to the room where the husband of our dead patient was waiting, I thought of giving Daniela some advice for the conversation we were about to have.

But just as there was no way to tell someone that they have cancer while preserving their smile, there was no way to be involved in such an uncomfortable conversation without feeling some of that discomfort oneself. There was no tip I could share or trick I could teach that would protect her.

In medical school we were taught to break bad news with mnemonics and flowcharts, no differently than how we are taught subjects like anatomy or physiology ("SPIKES—A Six-Step Protocol for Delivering Bad News," one such acronym is titled). I have found these frameworks to be tremendously useful when they are deployed correctly. They apply research and theory to help us develop a mental road map to navigate these difficult conversations.

Nevertheless, these tools cannot prepare us for the discomfort that such circumstances necessitate. Moreover, I sometimes worry that the existence of these frameworks can suggest that there is a single best way to deliver such news—that if a conversation does not go well, it is because the deliverer has failed to adhere well enough to the ideal framework of our protocols. As a result, when I teach them to medical students and residents, I worry that they might look upon these protocols not as the frameworks they are designed to be, but as scripts they are expected to follow. Too much focus on the specifics of such techniques can come at the expense of simply being present in the moment and understanding its significance. Such an approach can come off as sterile and meaningless, like a telemarketing script.

At this early stage in her career, I decided not to teach SPIKES to Daniela. The experience itself would be the lesson. We entered the room to speak with the husband.

TWELVE

AT LAST, AN INTRODUCTION

Before we even said a word, the husband approached us. "Thank you for everything you guys did. Everyone. The whole team. Thank you."

Grieving family members are almost universally appreciative, and yet it is a terrible feeling to be thanked by those who have lost the most. Their appreciation is difficult to accept. One cannot help but think, *No, no, we did a lot for all the* other *patients in the emergency room tonight. But it was your wife alone for whom we could not do enough.* Their appreciation transforms into our guilt.

I responded, "Oh, no need to thank us, this is why we are here. I'm sorry that we couldn't have done more."

We sat down. I had two goals for this conversation. In one I would have to provide information, and in the other I would do my best to obtain information.

First, it was critical to explain everything that had happened in the previous hours. From being at home with his wife, to watching her receive chest compressions while being loaded in an ambulance, to hearing her pronounced dead in the emergency room, my patient's husband had just witnessed a barrage of intense activity within a short period of time. As he would try to make sense of his day, it would be important for him to understand the rationale behind the actions that the paramedics and our emergency room team took.

Second, I needed to try to obtain some more information from him. After all, despite so much of consequence having occurred, I still knew very little about my patient. She had died under my care, yet I did not even know her name. If I were able to get some more information, I hoped, then perhaps I could gain some insight into the actual cause of her death. Anything that could make the situation less of a mystery would be a step forward both for our team and for the husband.

I started.

"Again, I'm very sorry for everything that happened today. I can't begin to understand what you must be going through. I know that so much has happened so quickly." I paused. "I'm hoping that if we talk for a bit, we can both get a better understanding of everything that took place."

He nodded understandingly and moved his lips ever so slightly as if wanting to say something, although no words came out.

"Before we begin, though, I realized that through all the commotion I never got the chance to truly introduce myself. My name is Dr. Nahvi. Farzon is my first name. Along with everyone else you saw today, I was taking care of your wife. And this is Daniela. She is on her way to becoming a doctor and is part of the team as well."

"Thank you very much," he replied, acknowledging us both. "I'm Anthony."

"Anthony, could you please tell me what your wife's name was before we go on?"

"Lola. Her name was Lola."

As we spoke, we switched between tenses—from present, to past, to present again. Lola's body had not yet been wheeled away. She was still there right beside us. The four of us inhabited the same space, yet we spoke about ourselves in the present tense while we spoke of her in the past.

"Thank you. I'm so sorry that I had to meet you and Lola under these circumstances."

Of course, one could dispute whether Lola and I had actually met today. Before, she was another limp, dead body. Now she was Lola. She had a presence.

I continued.

"I know you were with Lola for most of the day and I believe that you were the one who called 911 on her behalf, is that right?"

He nodded once more.

"So why don't you tell me what you know up until this point and then I'll pick it up and fill you in on what I know after that. Does that work?"

"Yes, of course . . . Where do I begin? Like I was saying earlier, we had come back from Florida last week. Everything was fine. Totally fine. But then two days ago she started to complain of some belly pain, but it was nothing that bad. I asked her if she wanted to go to the ER then, but she said no. She thought it was just gas or something she ate. I convinced her to at least make an appointment with her doctor—the appointment is for tomorrow actually . . ." He trailed off. "I guess we're not going to need that," he said, looking away briefly.

He paused, collecting himself. That her appointment still existed while she no longer did seemed to drive his new reality home.

He continued.

"Anyway. Earlier today her belly pain got real bad and then she began having some chest pain, too. She's not much of a complainer and I've never seen her like that in my life. She *still* didn't want to come to the ER, but I just went ahead and called 911 for her anyway. And that's pretty much it."

I picked up where he left off.

"Well, when the paramedics got to the emergency room they told me pretty much everything you just told me, so that is what I heard as well. They told me that when they showed up, Lola was in a good amount of pain but that she otherwise looked well. But then they said that she started complaining of some shortness of breath in addition to her abdominal and chest pain and it was at that point that she collapsed. Does all that sound about right?"

"Yeah . . . Yes."

"Was she having any shortness of breath before that point? Or was that just in the moments before she collapsed?"

"I don't think so. She was only complaining of pain in her stomach and her chest to me until the paramedics got there."

"And she wasn't complaining of any palpitations, any light-headedness, any fevers, or any pain or swelling in her legs, or anything else at all?"

"No, nothing. She was really just complaining mostly of some stomach pain."

"And your trip was just to Florida, right? You didn't leave the country before that or go anywhere else?"

"Yeah, we were just at a wedding in Miami. That's all."

"And she had no medical problems herself? No surgeries in the past? She wasn't taking any medications every day for any reason?"

"No. Nothing. She took care of herself."

"Do you have any idea if anyone in Lola's family had died at a young age, by any chance? I'm just trying to see if anything might have run in her family."

"I can't be sure, but, no—I don't think so."

"Okay, I'm sorry for all the questions. I'm just trying to get a better idea of what could have happened. To be honest, it's still pretty difficult to say." I continued. "What I heard from the paramedics was that after she collapsed, they checked her pulse and noticed that she didn't have one. What that tells us is that whatever was going on was pretty serious. Due to whatever problem she was having—whatever was causing her abdominal pain and chest pain and her shortness of breath—it caused her heart to effectively stop."

Early on in my career, I was often concerned about speaking down to patients. I worried that if I said things like "her not having a pulse tells us that something very serious was happening," it could be interpreted as some sort of an insult.

Of course not having a pulse is serious, you idiot, I would imagine them thinking.

Nevertheless, I quickly learned that this was almost never the case. The mindset of a person receiving such heavily loaded information is quite different from their mindset in any other circumstance. Any information we provide can quickly become overwhelming. No matter what we say or how we say it, family members often ask us to slow down and repeat what we have told them. I have come to appreciate that far from feeling talked down to, family members in such circumstances seem to like it when we speak in simple, repetitive terms.

"I also want you to know that the paramedics who were with your wife—their names are Winston and Lewis—they're two of the best we work with. She couldn't have been in better hands."

It was becoming clear that we were unlikely to have any clean answers for what caused Lola's death today. From everything that Anthony told me, there was nothing definitive that could guide us toward any one explanation. This is not unusual. Working in the emergency room, it is not uncommon for patients to arrive already dead, already undergoing CPR by the paramedics. As their hearts have already stopped pumping, we cannot perform an EKG to see if they had died from a potential heart attack. With their lungs no longer exchanging air, it is not the time to obtain a chest x-ray to diagnose a possible respiratory issue. And because they are unable to speak with us to tell their story, we cannot ask what they were feeling in the moments before they fell to the ground. Many times we never learn what, precisely, led to our patients' collapse.

As it was increasingly apparent that I would not be able to provide Anthony with the comfort of any answers, I thought that it would be important for him to at least be free of any second-guessing about the quality of care his wife received.

"Winston and Lewis immediately did all the right things and they did a great job. They started CPR, they gave her some fluids through the IV, they quickly placed a breathing tube in her. They also gave her a medication called epinephrine that can sometimes help the heart start beating again. They did everything they needed to do and they brought her to us as quickly as they could."

I wanted to reassure Anthony that he did everything *he* could have done as well, and that in addition to feeling at ease with the care his wife received, he should not have to second-guess himself, either.

Given that Lola had been feeling unwell for two days before she died, however, I was unconvinced that this was actually true. It's very likely there was in fact a reasonable chance that more could have been done had Lola arrived at the emergency room sooner. Whatever had been happening in her body had been developing for some time before it finally attacked. Quite possibly, I thought, if Lola or Anthony had called an ambulance or she had otherwise received medical care at an earlier stage, she might still be alive right now.

I wondered whether there was any benefit in telling Anthony any of this. I recalled a scenario where I was once forced to torture a patient's family member in such a way.

This family member was in her late twenties. She had been out at a restaurant having dinner with her father, when, in the middle of their meal, he was struck with a sudden change in his speech. While they had been conversing fluently only moments earlier, he suddenly began having a great deal of difficulty gathering his thoughts and expressing his words. He spoke haltingly and took his time pronouncing his words. He was mostly unintelligible. She suggested that they go to the emergency room. He dismissed her. They continued to eat.

They paid their bill, left the restaurant, and parted ways. She told me later that her father was a stubborn man and, as he had already refused to seek medical attention, she decided that she would let him "sleep it off." It was not until two days later, when his symptoms did not improve, that she ignored his continued resistance to the emergency room, picked him up from his home, and drove him to the hospital.

He had, of course, suffered a stroke. The portion of his brain responsible for his ability to communicate language had been deprived of the oxygen it needed to function. As brain damage caused by a lack of oxygen is largely irreversible, there was a good chance that he would sputter, stutter, and mumble his way through the remainder of his life.

It would be easy to criticize their decision to delay their emergency room visit—of course a stroke should be evaluated immediately, one might think. Yet it was clear that both patient and daughter were full of good intentions. What is obvious to one person may be ambiguous to another.

When this patient finally did arrive at the emergency room, we identified his stroke but had little to offer him. Depending on a variety of factors, strokes can be treated only within the first four and a half to twenty-four hours after the onset of symptoms. After that, we can offer physical therapy and rehabilitation to help patients adjust to their deficits and cross our fingers for some improvement, but we have nothing to reverse the damage that has already been done.

As things began to settle, this patient's daughter came over to me with a particularly difficult question. She asked me if she had made a mistake by not bringing him to the emergency room sooner. She asked me if she should have ignored her father and brought him to the emergency room over his refusals, during their dinner when his symptoms began. She asked me if things would have been different if she did.

Of course, what happened was not her responsibility. The patient himself had refused medical attention. One cannot be blamed for not taking stronger action to help someone against their own expressed wishes. Nevertheless, she was a caring family member of someone who had just suffered a serious debility. It became obvious that she was already beginning to take personal responsibility for what had occurred.

I told her that she did the best she could with the information that she had at the time. I told her that what constitutes an emergency is difficult to predict in real time and that her situation was made even tougher given that her father was refusing to come to the emergency room.

Nevertheless, I also knew that patients who suffer one stroke are at high risk for suffering subsequent strokes. And as mentioned, the medications and interventions we use to treat a stroke are effective only if they are administered within a few short hours of the onset of symptoms. "Time is brain," the old saying goes. Indeed, our true responsibility at this point was not to treat his current stroke, but to do what we could to minimize his chance of having subsequent strokes down the line. Ensuring that this patient and his family members had a solid understanding of how to identify and act on stroke symptoms, then, was an essential part of the medical care we were obligated to provide. It felt important for this patient's daughter to know that, should similar symptoms reoccur, she should rush her father to the emergency department. Things could indeed be different if quicker actions are taken.

"It doesn't make a difference for this visit," I told her. "We're going to do whatever we need to do to make sure he recovers as best he is able to now that this has happened. But if something like this ever happens again, then yes, you should not wait and you should bring him in right away. We do have some treatments for strokes, but we can only administer them if patients arrive quickly."

I gave her information that it was essential for her to know—indeed, she had asked for it. Nevertheless, for the rest of that evening, I cringed as I walked by this patient and his daughter. Sitting by his bedside through the night, she rocked herself back and forth. "Daddy, I'm sorry I waited. I fucked up, I'm sorry I waited, I didn't know, Daddy," I overheard her tell him as tears dripped down her face.

Recalling this, I wondered how much I should tell Anthony. Like the stroke patient, Anthony's wife may indeed have had a very different outcome had Anthony and Lola not waited so long to call 911.

And yet theirs was a very different circumstance. Unlike the stroke patient, there was no "next time" I needed to prepare Anthony for. Unlike the stroke patient, this did not feel like a teachable moment. Furthermore, I could not be completely certain that we would have had a treatment for Lola had she come in earlier, as I was still unsure what it was that actually caused her to die. There was little to be gained then, I reasoned, from suggesting that it was possible for her death to have been prevented. Thus, rightly or wrongly, I decided to keep my thoughts on the matter to myself. I gave no hint of my belief that there existed a scenario in which Lola would have survived.

"And thank you so much, Anthony, for calling 911 on her behalf. I know you said she didn't want you to, but I'm glad you did. It's never easy to know whether some little pain is going to turn out to be a big deal or turn out to be nothing at all. It's difficult to know when to make that call. You did everything you could have done and you gave her the best shot by calling the ambulance for her."

Somehow, the words I spoke simultaneously felt disingenuous and entirely appropriate.

He offered nods of understanding.

I continued my explanation of the day's events.

"Despite everything we did, we couldn't identify anything specific. And from what you told me, there really wasn't anything new or unusual going on that could point us in any particular direction. So to be completely honest, it's still quite unclear what exactly happened." I paused. "But I know that I have talked a lot so far—do you have any questions for us right now?" I asked, including Daniela in the conversation.

He shook his head no.

Feeling unsettled by the quiet energy in the room, I felt the urge to keep talking. Nevertheless, I had nothing more to say. Saying anything would have simply been an effort to address my own discomfort.

I looked over at Daniela. Her initial eagerness to be involved seemed to have faded.

Finally, without a single word or even a twitch of a muscle, the atmosphere in the room changed. It felt as if it would be more appropriate to give Anthony some space.

"It looks like you might want some privacy. We're going to step out of the room, but we'll be around. Don't hesitate to grab one of us if you need something or if you just want to talk."

We walked out the room and quietly shut the door behind us.

THIRTEEN

THE ABSURDITY OF BUREAUCRATS

Walking back to the chaos of the emergency room, I was quickly reminded of all the miscellaneous tasks and duties that competed for my attention. The quiet anxiety of the room we had just exited seemed an entirely different universe from the urgent energy of the rest of the ER.

A clerk pointed me toward a death certificate to fill out. An overhead announcement notified me that the medical examiner was waiting on the phone. A nurse asked me to check a box to indicate whether Lola's body was destined for the morgue or the autopsy room. The bureaucratic demands of our job stand in stark contrast to its more human elements. When one has just walked a man through the slow internalization of the death of his wife, it is difficult to appreciate the value of check boxes, classification codes, and billing procedures. Compounding matters, the medical world seems to embrace a particularly absurd version of bureaucratic demands.

I recall a mandatory online course about sleep hygiene that I was once assigned to as a resident in training. Requiring its residents to work twenty-seven-hour shifts every third day for weeks on end, my hospital began to entertain the notion that such a workload might lead to bad outcomes for its patients. Rather than consider a more reasonable schedule, however, it had determined that its physicians needed to develop a better understanding of how sleep deprivation can affect their work performance.

I still vividly remember sitting up in my bed, the faint blue glow of my laptop straining my eyes, fighting off the urge to sleep in order that I could be taught about the virtues of getting rest.

This type of absurdity is not unique.

More than 90 percent of American emergency rooms routinely report crowded conditions.[1] Nurses and physicians are often tasked with caring for twice the number of patients that they could reasonably be asked to care for. Without the physical space in which to place them, patients often spill over into hallways, stacked on stretchers in public areas of the hospital without even a curtain to guard their privacy. More than a mere annoyance, this type of overcrowding is known to be dangerous—numerous studies have demonstrated a direct link between emergency room overcrowding and increases in patient mortality.[2,3] Nevertheless, it is common for institutional funds to be spent not on hiring more nurses and doctors in order to address this life-threatening danger, but on billboards, magazine advertisements, and posters plastered on subways and buses, all eagerly inviting

even more people to come to our already overcrowded facilities. We spend our finite resources not on solutions that
might decongest our emergency rooms and save our patients'
lives, but on marketing campaigns designed to attract yet
more people to hospitals that have already proven themselves
beyond their capacity to safely care for them.

Focused on billing codes, documentation levels, and op-
erational costs, those who run our hospitals sometimes seem
to forget about the oxygen saturations, blood pressures, and
heart rates that represent the ultimate point of our efforts.
They invest tremendous efforts to stabilize our institutional
vital signs, while, at the same time, they forget to invest in the
things that would prevent the vital signs of our patients from
deteriorating. It is not unusual for me to walk into my shifts
only to note that my hospital's buildings are in better shape
than many of my patients are.

For all the impossible situations we face in healthcare, it
is often where we have the most control—the very system in
which we administer healthcare—that we are most stunned
by what we see.

Once, while working in one of New York City's public
hospitals, I cared for a patient who arrived at my emergency
department requesting treatment for her ovarian cancer. She
told me that she already had a biopsy-confirmed diagnosis of
the disease, that she had received several rounds of chemotherapy, and that she had arrived in order to obtain a subsequent round. Confused, I explained to her that emergency
rooms are incapable of administering chemotherapy—that the
way to obtain chemotherapy would be to go to an oncologist

who would arrange such treatments for her in an office or in an infusion center, as an outpatient.

"But my oncologist told me to come here," she replied.

I had assumed there was a misunderstanding before she passed me a piece of paper. Under letterhead from an Ivy League medical center, it read: "Ms. Shute has been under my care for treatment of stage IIIC low grade serous carcinoma of the right ovary. She is status post optimal cytoreductive surgery and undergoing adjuvant chemotherapy with carboplatin and paclitaxel, currently on cycle 4 of 6. Due to a change in the status of her health insurance, she was unable to complete the remainder of her chemotherapy treatment with me. I have referred her to [your] Hospital for the continuation and completion of her oncological care. Please evaluate and treat."

Ms. Shute went on to tell me that she had previously had a steady job that provided her with reliable health insurance. She told me that while working at this job, she was diagnosed with ovarian cancer and that she had begun receiving treatments for her cancer at a nearby academic medical center. Despite having never previously used her sick days at her work, she had exceeded her limit that year as a result of her cancer treatments. Because of this, she said that she was fired from her job, and as a result of that, she lost her health insurance as well. After she lost her health insurance, the oncologist who had been caring for her had informed her that she would no longer be able to obtain care at her facility. In effect, Ms. Shute told me that she had lost her ability to obtain medical care for her cancer precisely because she had been diagnosed with it.

Still, I was confused by her arrival at the emergency room.

Lacking both the tools and expertise to provide her with any cancer therapy, I asked her why her oncologist told her to go to the emergency room rather than make an appointment in one of our hospital's clinics.

"She didn't. She just told me to go to your hospital but she never said where to go or when to show up or anything. I wasn't sure where to go but I assumed I should come to the emergency room because I don't have insurance and I thought that there was a law that emergency rooms have to treat you if your condition is life threatening."

I bristled as I began to realize that her arrival to the emergency room was neither mistake nor simple misunderstanding.

"Well, you're right," I started. "There is a law like that, but all it says is that anyone who walks into an emergency room has the right to be *stabilized*. I know you have cancer and that it's life threatening, but technically, because it's not life threatening at this moment, you would be considered stable right now. I know it sounds crazy. More importantly, though, it's not that I don't want to treat you, but that I can't: I don't have access to any chemotherapies and even if I did, I'm an ER doctor, not an oncologist—you wouldn't want me to administer chemotherapy any more than you'd want your oncologist to put in a breathing tube. It's not something I know much about. We just don't have the capability to treat cancer in an ER."

"Wait, so you're saying that the law says that if I'm dying *quickly*, then I am guaranteed to get treated in the emergency room, but that if I'm dying *slowly*, then all bets are off?"

The accuracy of her depiction of our healthcare system made me uncomfortable. "Well, kinda—but we're not—"

She interrupted.

"So you can't treat my cancer now, but if I went home and then in a few months I came back when the cancer that's killing me now was killing me *more*—like it was actually game over and I was actually about to close my eyes and die—*then* you could treat me?"

"I guess, yeah, if that happened and then you were unstable at that point, we would certainly do whatever we could to stabilize you. I mean, I still wouldn't be able to treat your cancer itself in the ER, but we would treat whatever other condition was going on at that time that was making you unstable. But look, we're not going to let any of that happen."

I explained that, as hard as it might have been for her to believe, in the context of American healthcare, she was actually in luck. I explained how, in most parts of the country, she might indeed have no options and nowhere else to turn, but that in New York City, there existed a robust system of public hospitals where she would be able to see an oncologist and continue to receive treatment for her cancer despite her lack of health insurance. "Don't worry, we'll be able to get you to where you need to be," I tried to reassure her.

"Sure," she said, seeming to not quite believe me.

I made the arrangements for her to follow up with an oncologist within our city's public hospital system. I explained that appointments were limited and because it would be difficult to obtain the details of what treatments she had obtained thus far, as those records were stored in a different hospital system's medical records, there might be a delay in her care and she might have to repeat some tests that she had already performed. "I know it's not ideal, but I think that it's the best we could do."

"Thanks," she replied, refusing to make eye contact.

When I was a medical student, many of my professors spoke about the sense of pride we would one day feel upon appreciating the awesome responsibilities that our profession entrusted us with. They never once mentioned the inverse. They never once mentioned the deep sense of shame we routinely feel in knowing that our profession lets so many of our patients down.

I wanted to apologize to Ms. Shute and call out our healthcare system. I wanted to explain that I understood how maddening her situation must have felt and that I was really trying to help—that, somehow, I was on her side and that I spend much of my free time outside of work advocating for precisely the kinds of healthcare reforms that would have prevented her from experiencing her exasperating circumstance to begin with. Trying to convince her that I was on her side just after walking her through the mechanics of how our system had manufactured her terrible state of affairs, however, felt somehow akin to a prison guard trying to convince an inmate that he personally thought our criminal justice system was unfair while escorting him back to his jail cell. From her perspective, I thought, I was part of the same system that had created her dilemma. I kept my thoughts to myself and discharged her from the emergency room.

Ms. Shute's experience is not unique. In the emergency

room we are frequent witnesses to our system's shortcomings. Often, we are left with even less agreeable outcomes.

Once, I cared for a patient who resorted to taking fish antibiotics purchased from a pet store after she could not afford to see a human doctor to obtain human antibiotics for her sore throat. Attempting to calculate the appropriate dose of antibiotics using instructions meant for minnows, this patient misjudged the appropriate amount and overdosed by an order of magnitude. As a result, she suffered severe neurological side effects, lost her balance, and fell down a staircase. In her attempt to avoid our system's costs, she ended up saddled with the expense of a stay in the intensive care unit.

I called our local poison control center to report her case. The city's toxicologists compile data on overdoses and poisonings so that they can better protect the public. I told the toxicologist on the other end of the line about what had occurred. "You're never going to believe this," I said, "but the patient took antibiotics from a pet store."

"I'm guessing fish antibiotics, right?" he responded, clearly believing me.

"Yeah, exactly. How'd you know?"

"It's almost always fish antibiotics. Most people who can get their hands on dog or cat antibiotics do okay but you need a prescription from a vet for those. You can get fish antibiotics over the counter from any pet store. They actually work if you can dose it right, but the problem is that they come in packets that need to be dissolved into huge tanks, so they're very strong and concentrated. It's really hard to get the dose right for a person, so it's not uncommon for people to mess it up. We see this a lot—whenever people overdose on pet antibiotics, it's almost always the fish formulation. If your patient can't afford to see a doctor, she's better off trying to get dog or cat antibiotics next time. We don't see a lot of problems with those."

On nearly every shift I work, I see patients who suffer from uncontrolled blood pressure and elevated blood sugar. They casually describe how they halve their insulin doses and space out their high blood pressure pills, taking them not as their doctors prescribe but as their wallets allow. Understanding the long-term consequences—knowing that skipping these medications puts them at higher risk for heart attacks and strokes, blindness and kidney failure, even toe and foot amputations—they tell me that they have no choice. And so, unable to afford their expenses, these patients get priced out of their hearts and minds, eyes and kidneys, feet and toes.

I have even seen patients forced to barter diseases for one another. I once cared for a young man who had recently been evaluated, diagnosed, and treated for a fractured wrist. Upon receiving the bill for that visit, he began experiencing chest pain, shortness of breath, palpitations, and a tingling around his tongue and lips. He had received the bill for his broken wrist only to have it precipitate a panic attack. Responsible for coming up with thousands of dollars he did not have, he ended up back in the emergency room. Our healthcare system had, quite literally, treated one illness only to create another.

The reality of our healthcare system is often difficult to digest. It is after years of accumulating experiences like these, then, that I have developed a certain aversion to the bureaucratic demands of life in the emergency room. One cannot help but develop a certain callousness toward a system that is itself so callous toward the very people it is supposed to serve.

The current task before me was to document my encounter with Lola. Starting with the template that Daniela, our emergency room scribe, had created, I would finalize a note that would mark the details of Lola's final moments into her medical record. Had she survived, the note would have served as a vital tool to communicate her medical course to the other physicians and nurses who would later care for her. Doctors and nurses rely on these notes to understand what previously happened to a patient in order to guide their care going forward. Often, an understanding of the past provides a blueprint for the future. Because Lola had died, however, the document would serve mostly as a record of our events.

I was aware, however, that this was not the only purpose for which our note would be used. Once they arrived at their offices in the morning, my hospital's billers and coders would extract our note from our hospital's computer system. Sitting in offices located in buildings that are a world away from the clinical environment in which we work, they would apply sophisticated software that would scour it for its most profitable phrases. Then, using a sort of free market alchemy, they would turn these words into revenue. "Strive to five" is a mantra of this process—a playful phrase that our billers and coders use to emphasize the importance of reaching a level five billing code, the most profitable one in an emergency room.

Ultimately, these billers and coders would generate not a

condolence letter, but a bill. They would first mail it to Lola's health insurance company, who would pay whatever portion of it they felt they were responsible for. The remainder of the bill—a copay, a coinsurance, a deductible, or any other amount that her insurance company refused to cover—would be mailed to Lola's home. Despite her death, Lola's estate— the legal term our hospitals' financial services departments use to refer to the economic valuation of Lola's assets, investments, and interests that remained after she had died—would be responsible for the remainder of the charges. Only if it was proven that Lola's life's savings had been depleted and there was no money left to pay, would the remainder of the hospital charges be written off and forgiven.

Of course, since she was dead, Anthony would check the mail one day only to find a letter in the name of his dead wife. He would open it and discover, perhaps, a statement itemizing thousands of dollars in charges for care that did not save her.

I wish this wasn't happening!, my brain howled once again as I sat at my computer to chronicle my encounter with Lola.

Death causes us discomfort by reminding us of the humanity we share. Our healthcare system's handling of death, on the other hand, causes us discomfort by reminding us of the shared humanity we choose to ignore.

As I documented the encounter, I sighed and clicked "sign," filing my note into the electronic medical record, aware of the sequence of events that would follow it.

FOURTEEN

CAUSE OF DEATH: ?

My next task was to fill out the paperwork required to report Lola's death to the local agencies. Unlike our hospitals, the medical examiner does not bill our patients or send them to collections agencies. So while dealing with them was also a morbid and bureaucratic task, it was a welcome shift.

I sat down to log in to the website run by the New York City Office of the Chief Medical Examiner. It is a database where every death that takes place in a city of eight million people is reported. Countless episodes of heartbreak are ultimately recorded as blips in a single enormous directory. The website loaded, but I could not proceed. I had forgotten my password. After several failed log-in attempts I was prompted for a reset. After several failed attempts at that—too many similarities to a prior password or too few special characters— I was finally granted access.

That I must go through the same circuitous process on a

web browser to record something as significant as a human death as I do to order more snack bites for my dog gives me pause. One feels as if profound events should be treated specially, outside of our normal workflows.

But this is not the case. While recording a birth or a death is infinitely more consequential than ordering some treats for my dog, there is no fundamental difference between either workflow on the back end. We use the same operating systems, markup codes, and usernames and passwords. If anything, the website where I order my dog's treats is better designed and more technologically advanced than the website I go to in order to tally a human life. The digital version of the pearly gates feels about two decades outdated.[1]

I was able to quickly fill out the time and date, my medical license number, and Lola's demographic information. I was forced to pause, however, when I came across a question that I remained unable to answer.

"Cause of death" the system prompted.

I have no idea, I thought.

This database was designed many decades ago for a very different environment from the emergency room. It was originally constructed for the medical and surgical wards, the inpatient side of the hospital.

Inpatient teams often have days, sometimes even weeks, to get to know patients and their medical problems. In the emergency room, on the other hand, we routinely lack this information. We often know nothing about our patients except that they have arrived. We can usually estimate their age within a decade or so and are mostly able to guess their gender. We may be able to assume they have heart disease by the footlong sternotomy scar on their chest, or we may predict that they are a dialysis patient by the bumpy fistula they wear over a bicep. But beyond reading into these types of observations, there is plenty of guesswork. Are those track marks on their arm a sign of intravenous drug use? Or was this person just at their doctor's office getting blood drawn for some recent and relevant illness? Is that chipped front tooth a sign that they fell and hit their head? Or did they simply suffer the misfortune of chomping on an olive pit years ago?

If patients arrive without a family member, a driver's license in their wallet, or some other sort of way to identify them, we assign something to call them by. Rather than refer to them with the ambiguity of "that patient that just showed up," we give them a name. The specific pseudonym we assign differs from hospital to hospital. Some hospitals refer to unknown patients in precisely that way: "Unknown Female 1" or "Unknown Male 4," with a higher number indicating, perhaps, a more hectic evening. Other hospitals get creative. "Trauma Texas" and "Trauma Oklahoma" were among the pseudonyms that were assigned at one hospital I previously worked at.

Of course, I had only recently learned Lola's name. Even after speaking with her husband, I still lacked enough information to identify what caused her death. Still, I knew that bureaucracies, like death itself, lie beyond one's ability to appeal.

"This field cannot be left blank," the red text warned beside the unanswerable question.

This, of course, is not unusual. In our attempt to control

life, we have created a litany of strict definitions and inflexible rules. We routinely codify and organize the events of our lives in order to ensure that they fit into the rigid structures we have created. Often, we go too far. We compartmentalize our lives beyond reason and we demand organization and answers where none may exist. We exchange meaningful experience for feckless information just to feed our algorithms. Ultimately, in doing this, we might succeed at controlling life only at the expense of losing its very essence.

Nevertheless, our system would not budge. I would have to venture a guess.

"Abdominal pain," I entered, the vagueness of my answer allowing for the preservation of my honesty.

Benny, our clerk, looked over my shoulder and laughed. "C'mon, dude, you know the system isn't going to accept that." Benny was tasked with processing the death certificate. Despite having never pronounced a patient's death, he was far more experienced with these forms than anyone else in the emergency room. Since the database would not listen to me, I made my appeal to him instead.

"Yeah, but I have no idea what the cause of death for this lady is. She literally arrived dead and all I know is that she had abdominal pain and chest pain at home. It could have been almost anything."

Sympathetic though he may have been, that changed nothing. He laughed once again. "You know the deal, you still have to write something. You just gotta fill it out."

"Cardiac arrest." I sighed as I typed.

It was a justifiable answer. Technically, every death is

ultimately "due" to cardiac arrest. After all, "cardiac arrest" is nothing more than medical jargon for "the heart has stopped." Cardiac arrest is, in a way, both a cause of death and the definition of it.

"Enter a proximal cause of death," the system requested.

The database was requesting a secondary diagnosis to explain what, precisely, *led* to the patient's cardiac arrest. Given that my previous response was vague to the point of being meaningless, it was a fair point.

"Cardiac arrest due to . . ." I thought out loud as I tapped my pen on the computer monitor, perhaps hoping someone else would finish my sentence. Kept hostage by the question— I could not proceed until the system was satisfied—I decided to take a look through Lola's lab results for any clues.

With every critical or unstable patient who is whisked to the emergency room we place an intravenous line and draw blood immediately upon their arrival. Their blood work, however, provides us with no immediate assistance. Blood tests take time to be sent to the laboratory, spun in their centrifuges, and undergo their analyses with photometers and flow cytometry machines. Our patients do not have the luxury of that time. These laboratory specimens are sent off, then, not to help guide our immediate resuscitation in the emergency room, but with the hope that their results could help to guide their care later, should our patient survive the initial critical moments. In other words, if our patients live long enough to make it to the intensive care unit, the blood tests that we have drawn in the emergency room help to inform the management that the critical care team will later provide in the ICU.

For Lola, who was pronounced dead before the lab results had ever returned, these results were nothing more than a formality. Because they served no functional purpose, I had failed to check them. Still, I thought, they might help with the paperwork. Perhaps an extraordinarily high white blood cell count might point to an infection, or an extremely low hemoglobin level would indicate that some sort of anemia was to blame. The lab results had finally begun to trickle back. I clicked a tab marked "Results Review."

It was then that I noticed a red exclamation point, indicating an abnormal result. It appeared beside the column for Lola's pregnancy test. Normally, I roll my eyes at the idea that our electronic medical record classifies pregnancy as an "abnormal result." This time, however, I agreed with the computer. Lola's pregnancy hormones were quite low, but they were beyond any ambiguous threshold.

Everything snapped into place. The most likely cause of Lola's death immediately became clear. Known as an ectopic pregnancy, Lola had gotten pregnant, but the pregnancy had implanted somewhere outside of the uterus, where it belongs. While the uterus is designed to expand and accommodate a growing fetus, other organs are not. And so, as the tiny embryo inside her had grown, it pushed against whatever structure it had mistakenly implanted beside, causing it to stretch and strain, explaining the two days of vague abdominal pain that Lola had had. Finally, unable to stretch any further, the structure burst, causing Lola to bleed out internally, explaining her shortness of breath, her chest pain, and ultimately, her collapse.

"All bleeding eventually stops," the surgical saying goes. Lola's bleeding had stopped not because it had become controlled and corrected, however, but because her body had simply run out of blood.

This was only a working hypothesis, but it was a pretty good one. Young and healthy people do not die for no apparent reason. Unexpected findings are generally not red herrings, but answers. My patient had abdominal pain, an unexpected pregnancy, and she died suddenly. Occam's razor sharpened and I suddenly felt quite confident of the cause of her death. Nevertheless, my "aha" moment was not a joyous one.

I remembered how Anthony phrased his response when I had asked him earlier, in the chaos of her resuscitation, if there was any chance that Lola might be pregnant. He said that he and his wife had tried to get pregnant but "couldn't." In a cruel twist of fate, the very thing that this couple wanted to happen but found themselves unable to achieve had finally happened. And it caused Lola to die.

Entering the field of emergency medicine, I was promised a career that would expose me to "a wide array of challenging and fulfilling experiences." Years later, I never considered that one day I would have to explain to a newly widowed husband how the unborn baby he did not know he had had just killed his wife.

FIFTEEN

KNOWLEDGE IS POWER.
IGNORANCE IS BLISS.

When information is truly agonizing, the fine line between "knowledge is power" and "ignorance is bliss" narrows. Which side of this divide we land on can depend on two factors: first, how agonizing the bit of information is, and second, the amount of power we have to affect the situation at hand. Sometimes we want to know right away—other times, we may prefer to be kept in the dark for a while.

As a resident in training, I gave no consideration to the notion that knowledge can be anything but power. A favorite part of my job has always been getting to know my patients' stories. It was their stories that enriched my job and kept me going. As I learned to set bones and stitch up wounds, I thrived on learning the anecdotes behind the injuries.

This process of listening to patients is in part a necessary component of our jobs. We need these stories in order to provide our patients with the appropriate medical treatments. I cannot correctly care for a patient's finger laceration, for example, unless I know whether that person was cut by a clean kitchen knife or by the jagged edge of a raw oyster shell. I cannot correctly care for my patient who presents with an animal bite unless I know whether they were bitten by their family's pet Chihuahua, or by a raccoon in the yard as they were taking out the trash. The right thing to do—whether antibiotics should be prescribed or a rabies injection administered, for example—depends on the stories behind the injuries. It is thus important to know what our patients were cooking for dinner and whether or not they have any pets.

But part of the pleasure of our job comes from going one step beyond this basic requirement and learning about our patients themselves. Who they are, what they are like, and how they perceive the world.

My affinity for patient stories is not unique—most physicians report that their patients are the primary source of fulfillment and satisfaction they receive from their work.[1] And as society's medical front porch, the emergency room is the ideal vantage point from which to witness the breadth of the experiences people may have. From philanthropists born into large inheritances to undocumented housekeepers who work hard for their pay, people from all walks of life are wheeled into the emergency room. We have the luxury of learning from all of them. And just as learning more about one's favorite musician somehow makes listening to their music more enjoyable, my job treating patients becomes richer as I learn more about them.

Of course, the majority of patient stories are rather ordinary.

KNOWLEDGE IS POWER. IGNORANCE IS BLISS.

While we may occasionally come across something unusual like a skydiving injury or an encounter with a dominatrix gone wrong, the vast majority of visits to the emergency room arise from the mundane. We see far more visits for abdominal pain caused from constipation than we do gunshot wounds and stabbings. Nevertheless, it is within these mundane stories that we find the deeper purpose to our jobs. After all, setting a broken bone or stitching up a wound with no human context behind it can eventually begin to feel like factory work—mindlessly functional and routine. That same broken bone or laceration, however, when injected with a background story, comes to life. A fractured ankle resulting from a drunken fall down three steps, for example, can grow boring and even elicit a silent reprimand (*Don't drink so much! You'll get hurt!*).

But learning that that same septuagenarian patient who fell down the stairs and broke her ankle was drunk because she was at a Sunday brunch with her college roommates, for example, elicits a far different reaction. This information may not help me treat her ankle fracture, but it changes how I feel about it. With just a few additional details, judgments fade and understanding develops. Now I might think, *Well, please be careful, but I'm glad you were out enjoying life with your friends.* These stories transform the healing profession from a robotic job to a human endeavor.

Even life-threatening situations can become endearing after they stabilize. I once cared for a six-year-old boy with a history of allergic reactions to pistachios. His mother had rushed him in for just that. His face had puffed up and he had hives throughout his body. He had mentioned that he had some difficulty breathing. The situation was concerning at first. Yet as he improved and his mother's panic faded, he began to tell us his version of the story. It became difficult to hold back a smile.

He told us that he knew he was not allowed to eat pistachios, but that, very simply, he wanted to do so anyway. "I really like pistachios a lot," was the totality of his justification for doing what he knew he was not allowed to do. When he found out that a friend had a bag of pistachios, he traded the snacks his mother had packed him for a handful of the nuts.

Making piercing eye contact and with an unmistakable defiance in his voice, his admission did not come with any hint of regret. He seemed unconcerned about his own health. I held back from asking the question I truly wanted to know his answer to: "Was it worth it?"

I wanted to ask mainly because I suspected that his answer would be "yes." The boy exuded the spirit of an adventurer— *Of course it was worth it. What is life for if not living?* I imagined him saying.

Several years into my career, however, I began to wonder whether all of these patient stories were worth hearing. For as much as the heartwarming stories uplifted, the cold and soggy stories bore down. Feeling the weight of these stories, powerless in their presence, I began to ask myself, *What is the point?* I began to wonder if I even wanted to hear some of them at all.

I once cared for a patient whose story started challenging my assumptions. This patient was unsheltered, living in the streets, subways, and parks of New York City. Drinking a gallon of hard liquor every day, he suffered from an alcohol use disorder—a disease that is often the cause *and* the consequence of living an unsheltered life. The unfortunate reality is that homeless patients suffering from alcoholism are not uncommon in New York City's emergency rooms. While the vast majority of New York's unsheltered population do not suffer from alcoholism or frequent the emergency room, many who suffer from alcoholism do show up often.

These patients commonly do not arrive of their own free will, but are brought in by paramedics or police officers after they are found drunk and unresponsive on a park bench or in a subway car. Sometimes the police are called because someone has reported a disturbance. Other times, a homeless patient sleeping on a subway car is enough to land them in the hospital.

This particular patient was well known to the staff of my emergency room. Browsing through his electronic medical record, one could see that he had accumulated daily visits, and on many days he would arrive multiple times. Reading the time stamps, I noted that many of his visits were often only hours apart from one another. Reading through some of the notes that my colleagues had written, it appeared that his visits would play out, more or less, from the same script.

Often this patient would be found intoxicated, slumped over on the street, at which time a concerned bystander would call an ambulance on his behalf. When the paramedics arrived, they would load him onto a stretcher and then onto their truck. Arriving at the emergency room triage station, someone would check his vital signs and monitor his blood glucose.[2] After being wheeled back to the core of the emergency room, this patient would then be seen by a physician, who would comb through his hair with gloved hands, feeling for any bumps or step-offs and checking for any fresh blood that could indicate a recent fall.[3] If no wounds were identified, this patient would then be awakened from his drunken slumber in order that we could ask him what happened that caused him to be brought to the emergency room. He would be asked if there was anything we could do for him. Having gone through the motions many times and well aware of our sequence of events, he would often reply with a single word. Shouting "Vodka!" he would communicate that he had merely been drinking vodka and that nothing else was bothering him. He knew what we wanted to know and knew that the sooner he informed us that he was merely drinking and that he had no other injury or ailment, the sooner we would allow him to go back to sleep. After he had rested for the three to four hours it took for him to sober up, we would awaken him once more. We would check that his speech was coherent and that he was steady on his feet. Determining him to be "clinically sober," we would then discharge him back to the streets. Eventually, he would start drinking once more until another concerned Samaritan would call 911 upon finding him, once again, passed out and slumped over.

There are countless patients who live this sort of existence in New York City. We get to meet many of them. We learn their names and we often develop complicated relationships with them.

There was one patient, Mr. Render, who embodied the complexities of these relationships well. A daily visitor to our hospital, Mr. Render would often be wheeled into our emergency room strapped to an ambulance stretcher. Upon entering the emergency room, he would free his arms from the safety restraints, extend them out wide, and beam a broad-toothed smile. "Papa's home!" he would loudly exclaim to everyone and no one in particular. As with any beloved sitcom character, it became his catchphrase. In his arms, he often held a bouquet of crumpled flowers that he would hand to the first nurse that he saw. It was clear that Mr. Render felt comfortable in the emergency room. If he overheard another patient giving a nurse or a physician a hard time, he would defend those of us who worked there, often threatening the other patient in the process. Cursing at them he would yell, "These people are trying to help you. Now sit the fuck down!" As much as we did not want our patients engaging in altercations among themselves, we were appreciative of the sentiment.

But Mr. Render was unpredictable. He could be aggressive and, on more than one occasion, crossed the line. It was not unusual to see him, in his drunken stupor, lazily swing his fists at one or another of my coworkers. He had tried to strike me on more than one occasion. More often than not, he would apologize afterward. Other times, I would catch Mr. Render sitting alone and crying for what seemed to be no reason in particular. A nurse had once warned me to be careful around him. He told me that Mr. Render had spent over a decade upstate in prison for manslaughter and that I should not become too comfortable around him. I had no way of verifying the statement.

I never learned where the flowers Mr. Render would bring came from or why he always seemed to have a bouquet of them handy despite living in the streets. I always wondered whether, knowing that sooner or later someone would call 911 on his behalf and that he would be brought to the emergency room, Mr. Render intentionally kept a bouquet of flowers within arm's reach so that he could hand them to our nurses. On some weeks, given the unpredictable nature of an emergency room schedule, I would see Mr. Render more often than I would see my wife. Somehow I considered him an important part of my life. At the same time, however, I was wary of him.

We learn a lot from patients like Mr. Render. In fact, given the sheer difference in their life's experience compared to our own, we may learn the most from them. It is our unsheltered patients, the prisoners we care for, and those suffering from psychiatric illnesses that have provided me with some of my most eye-opening insights.

The patient who would speak to us with a one-word reply—"Vodka"—was no different. As is typical for patients living in the streets, he had lice in his hair and grime under his fingernails. He smelled exactly as one might expect him to smell. He wore multiple T-shirts, sweatshirts, and even multiple jackets—the innermost layers were crusted over and appeared not to have been removed in ages. His feet smelled like rotting flesh—largely because that is precisely what they were. His legs suffered from his diabetes and the changes of chronic venous stasis—the swelling that occurs as a result of years of sleeping in an upright seated position on a park bench or subway car—and his blood could no longer supply his legs with the nutrition their cells needed to survive. As a result, areas on his legs began to rot while still connected to his body. He did not yet have maggots growing in them as so many other patients in his condition did, but it seemed as if this were only a matter of time. He was the stereotypical unsheltered patient of New York—the type of patient who would cause me to scoff whenever I saw a homeless person portrayed on television or in a movie. A makeup artist could fake dirt under fingernails or imitate lice in a wig, but no actor could replicate the years of wear and toil that patients like him embodied.

I checked this patient's vital signs and his blood glucose in our computer system. They were normal. I went over to his bedside. Like many people in the emergency room who are alcohol dependent, he was sleeping comfortably when I arrived. I ran my gloved fingers through his hair, finding mites and nits but no blood or evidence of a skull fracture. I disturbed his slumber in order to ask him, as we ask all of our patients, what brought him to the emergency room that day. The computer record demonstrated hundreds of visits with nearly the same exact course of events, so I had a good guess for what it would be. Still, today might have been different—one always hopes that one day might be different for patients like these. And so, I asked.

When he awoke, he did not do so gently, rubbing his eyes and yawning, but shooting up, swinging his fists in the air in every direction. Many unsheltered patients, I have observed over the years, wake up instinctively throwing punches in the air. They frantically jolt their heads from side to side in search of whoever might have woken them. Sleeping on the streets, one is vulnerable. Everything is a threat. Consciousness demands a reflex to violence.

I asked him again what brought him to the emergency room. His only response, consistent with everything I had read in his electronic medical record, was "Vodka." Despite our standing next to each other, he shouted it. He was partially toothless. He smacked his lips and went back to sleep.

I allowed him to rest and thought little of the encounter as I went on to see some of the other patients waiting to be evaluated in the emergency room.

Hours later, upon reassessing him to ensure that he was steady on his feet and ready for discharge, I decided I would try again. I asked him how he was doing and what we could do for him. "Vodka, vodka," he replied once again, shaking his head and waving me away. I asked him if he felt better now that he had rested, and if there was anything else bothering him. Was he ready to leave? He nodded his head affirmatively. Before he left, however, I felt the urge on this day to ask him "Why?" Why was he drinking so much, every day, day after day? Was there anything we could do to help?

At first, he did not want to engage. He brushed me off again. I insisted and he resisted again. I told him I could help. Eventually he told me his story.

He said that he was an Afghan immigrant who had somehow ended up in New York City. He said he was a sniper back in Afghanistan. He pulled a pretend rifle to his cheek and mouthed the sounds of gunshots. He whipped his shoulder backward as if his imaginary rifle had a powerful recoil.

He told me that he killed countless Russians many years ago, and that, in more recent years, he killed countless Afghans as well. He told me that he had killed Americans, too.

He said, "Everyone is trying to kill me. I killed everyone. Now everyone is trying to kill me. Even God is trying to kill me with the vodka." His single-word answer suddenly seemed to mean much more.

He told me that his immediate family had died in Afghanistan. He once had a large extended family, he told me, but many of them had died as well. He told me that whenever he was sober, his only thought was to kill himself. The only way he could avoid his thoughts of suicide was to drink. And so he drank all day, every day, in order to keep living. He said that he believed that the type of life he was living was itself a form of death.

It was obvious that our usual protocol—providing him with some information on an alcohol cessation program for his drinking, a printed list of the nearest homeless shelters for his living situation, and a psychiatric evaluation for the suicidal thoughts he mentioned having—would be insufficient. Still, I did not know what else to do, so I offered them.

He laughed at my suggestions and then became angry that I invoked a psychiatrist. He demanded that I leave him alone. Ultimately, after his evaluation was complete, he was discharged.

I saw him again several more times over the coming weeks. Each time, I wondered what more I could provide for him. Yet there was nothing I could think to do, nothing I could provide, and nothing I could say that would create any substantive change.

Perhaps I was simply witnessing a limit to my creative thinking. Perhaps there was a solution that I failed to see.

Nevertheless, this patient had no interest in evaluating his drinking or considering that he stop. A psychiatrist had determined that he would not benefit from any inpatient evaluation for his suicidal thoughts. Claiming that the other residents at the city's shelters were unpredictable and dangerous and that the shelters themselves imposed too many restrictions and rules, the patient refused to entertain the idea of moving into a homeless shelter as well. He told me that he preferred the independence and freedom of the city's park benches and subway cars. He had no interest even in having a conversation. "You don't understand," was all he would tell me whenever I tried to talk to him. Then he would roll over in his hospital bed and turn his back toward me.

Over the next few years, I would see this patient every so often during one of my shifts. All of these interactions were similar to the ones that came before. He would arrive in the emergency room intoxicated. I would go over to wake him. I would duck his punches, review his vital signs and his blood sugar, and brush my fingers through his hair. I would ask him what brought him in. He would reply, "Vodka," I would give him a thumbs-up in understanding and would walk away, allowing him the time to sober up. Hours later, I would print his discharge papers and send him on his way.

The only real change that occurred as a result of my probing him for his story was that, now, upon bringing him his meals, I would bring him an extra sandwich or carton of milk, feeling sorry for his situation and not knowing what else I could do. Somewhere along the way, I wondered why I had insisted that he tell me his story at all. It felt, in a way, as if my insistence on this was somehow cruel. He told me that I wouldn't be able to help, that I should back off, and it seemed he was right.

His story caused me to retreat. For a time, I stopped asking my patients for extra details and I began to accept the bare minimum I needed to perform my job. If I feared an answer would only cause dismay and no opportunity to help, I held back from further questioning.

Of course, I knew that my change in approach was not an actual solution to his problem or any other. I knew that ignoring something because it was difficult to hear did not make it go away, and I was under no illusion that censoring my experience was the right thing to do. Very simply, however, I needed a break.

The experience allowed me to appreciate that while knowledge is power, it can also overpower. While some of us may prefer to enter a chilly pool by diving in headfirst, others need to dip their toes and ease their way in. We all have a threshold of what we can tolerate. In this way, some of us may prefer to experience bleak or overwhelming news all at once, while others need it delivered more slowly, taking time to process the information little by little.

I wondered what Anthony's preference might be.

Already devastated by the death of his wife, how would he take the news that Lola was pregnant when she died? How would he take the news that it was her pregnancy that killed her? Certainly, the information would be difficult to hear. And there was nothing he could do to affect the situation. What was his threshold? Would knowledge be power, or would he prefer to have remained ignorant of the truth I was about to tell him? There was no way to know.

The catch is that we cannot know what our threshold is until we exceed it. By then, of course, it is too late to turn back. Once we are exposed to information, it is impossible to unlearn it.

Ultimately, however, these questions were purely philosophical. My obligation was clear. I had important information that was essential to Anthony's understanding of his wife's death. I did not know how he would take it, but I had to tell him.

SIXTEEN

ON HOW TO REQUEST A DEAD PATIENT'S PERMISSION

I searched for Anthony so that I could speak with him once more. I found him back in Lola's room, staring at her and standing in the room in silence. He looked up at me as I walked in.

"Sorry to interrupt," I began. "I wanted to let you know that some of the results of the blood tests we ran came back and there's some more information that we learned about your wife. I wanted to go over it with you if that would be okay. Let me know when might be a good time to do that."

"Yes, of course. Now is fine," he said, as he slowly began to follow me out the door.

As I waited outside the room, I thought through what it would actually mean to divulge Lola's pregnancy to him. I had never encountered this particular scenario before. Anthony certainly had a right to know the cause of his wife's death. It would be unethical to keep that information from him. He also had at least some right to know that she was pregnant with his child—such information certainly affected him as well.

But there was more to it.

As part of our work, we do, on occasion, learn that a patient is incidentally pregnant. In the effort to ensure that pregnant patients do not experience unnecessary radiation from our CT scans and x-rays, for example, and to ensure that the medications we prescribe are not harmful to a potential fetus, we routinely perform pregnancy tests in the emergency room. Every so often, we end up with an unexpectedly positive result.

In normal circumstances, if we were to find a positive pregnancy test when our patient had actually arrived for a fever, for example, we would navigate the situation with intention. If such a patient had someone accompanying them, we would first return to that patient's room to ask that their companion step outside. Only then, when they are alone and in private, would we divulge the news of the positive pregnancy. After this is done we might then ask our patient if it would be okay to call their companion back into the room.

In the overwhelming majority of cases, this process is overkill. Patients often laugh at our delicate approach, finding it excessive when the person we ask to step out is their partner. "Of course you can tell him, he's the father," they might say.

There are circumstances, however, where a patient does not find our protocol to be exaggerated. These patients may ask us that we not inform their partner of the news. Before I spoke with Anthony, this thought crossed my mind.

It would have been ideal, of course, to simply ask Lola if I could tell Anthony that she had died because of her pregnancy. Based on my experience, the overwhelming odds were that she would want me to tell him. She would want her husband to know what caused her to die, so that he could have some answers, and, perhaps, some closure. Most likely she would want him to know that for however brief a period of time, she was pregnant with his child.

In the rare circumstances in which the pregnant woman does not want us to inform their partner, however, the situation can be fraught. These situations often stem from the delicate dynamics of an undesired pregnancy, infidelity, or domestic abuse. What if this was one of those circumstances?

What if Anthony did not know that his wife was pregnant, but she knew all along? After all, all of the information I knew about Lola, I had obtained from Anthony. What if Lola was aware she was pregnant, and had been refusing a visit to the doctor for her abdominal pain because she was planning on terminating her pregnancy? What if Lola knew she was pregnant, but that it was not Anthony's child? Would it be right not to tell a grieving husband the cause of his wife's death because of the slim but real chance that something like this was the case?

Once again we had entered a gray area. I was to navigate the situation without clear guidance from our ethics, principles, or norms.

With no definitive guidance, I recalled a previous patient case that helped inform me.

There was an elderly Greek woman I had cared for years ago. She spoke no English and had arrived at the emergency room accompanied by her daughter, who translated on her behalf. We are taught to avoid the use of friends or family members to serve as medical translators. If we have the capability, we are encouraged to use a neutral professional translator whenever possible. It is precisely for patient encounters like the one I was about to have that we do this.

I reached for a translator phone—a specialized telephone with two handsets, one of which is given to the patient and the other of which I hold up to my own ear. These phones dial a medical interpretation service that has the capability to translate dozens of languages and dialects. As I did this, however, I was waved away—instead, my patient pointed me toward her daughter. Figuring this was permission enough to hang up the phone and have the patient's daughter translate instead, I went along with it. In hushed and hurried tones, my patient's daughter began to tell me why she had brought her mother into the hospital.

"Okay, so my mom has ovarian c-a-n-c-e-r—don't say the word because she knows that word in English. She's been having pain because she has a lot of fluid in her belly because of the you-know-what. Her oncologist told us to come here to get it drained, so that's why we're here. We've already had to do this several times and she always feels a lot better afterwards, so we're just here to get the fluid drained and then we'll go home."

The procedure she was referring to is called a therapeutic paracentesis. Fluid can build up in the abdomen as a result of a variety of medical conditions. In patients with ovarian cancer, this fluid buildup is often due to the blockage of the lymph nodes that drain our body's fluids as well as a change in the proteins our body makes. As fluid fills in our patients' bellies faster than the skin that overlies it can stretch, the skin begins to feel tight like a drumhead, causing a constant and gnawing pain. The solution to this problem is straightforward: we drain the fluid. To do this, we insert a needle connected to some tubing into the abdomen, allowing the excess fluid to drain into a bag. Once the pressure is released, patients report immediate relief.

While I agreed that my patient would benefit from the procedure, I immediately became uncomfortable about performing it. I was being asked, it seemed, to perform an invasive medical procedure on a patient who was being kept in the dark about her illness. This patient may have lacked the ability to speak English, but she certainly retained her capacity to make decisions on her own behalf. Knowingly withholding a cancer diagnosis from a patient such as this would be an egregious violation of her autonomy. I could not, in good conscience, insert a needle into any patient without telling them why.

I told the daughter that the plan to drain the fluid in her mother's belly sounded reasonable, but that I would first want to speak with her myself to confirm everything. I went over to grab one of the handsets of the translator phone. She stood in my way and prevented me from reaching the phone.

"Listen, I don't want you to get on the phone with her because she *cannot* know that she has c-a-n-c-e-r. If you try to tell her she has c-a-n-c-e-r I'm taking her and we're leaving."

This patient's daughter was trying to get me to change my behavior by threatening her mother's health. She had leveraged our shared concern for her mother to get me to do what *she* thought was right.

It worked.

I put the phone down to consider my options.

She continued: "She'd be absolutely devastated if she found out. She wouldn't be able to handle it. Anyway, we've been treating her for a while now and nobody else has ever had a problem with it. You can check the notes in your computer system if you don't believe me."

I stepped out of the room to collect my thoughts and decide on an approach. I sat down at a computer terminal and took the daughter up on her suggestion. Browsing through my patient's health records, I was surprised to learn that the daughter's story was, in fact, confirmed. According to the notes from the patient's oncologist and from her prior visits to have the fluid in her abdomen drained, it appeared that she had been receiving treatment for her cancer without her having any knowledge of the disease. She had even received chemotherapy, it seemed, and was never informed of her cancer diagnosis.

Increasingly uncomfortable with the situation, I decided that I would call the patient's oncologist to get a better understanding. I dialed the number we had on file. Without a secretary or answering service, he immediately picked up the phone. I introduced myself and indicated that I was calling on behalf of "Ms. P with the ovarian cancer—" He cut me off.

"Ah yes, thank you for calling. I sent her in for a therapeutic paracentesis," he said. "Her belly is getting big again and it's making her very uncomfortable. I was hoping you could help her out for me. She's a very nice lady and a dear friend of mine." He had a thick Greek accent himself. He sounded experienced.

I asked about her apparent lack of awareness of her diagnosis.

"Ah yes, her family thought it would be better if she didn't know. She's very old and it would crush her to find out."

I remained silent.

"In Greek culture, cancer is *very* bad," he went on to say, as if there existed any culture in which cancer was not. "It has a bad *stigma*." He pronounced the world "stigma" slowly and emphasized its vowels. It was the product of his accent, yet it somehow gave the impression that he harbored a special respect for the word. "But she has a good family and they are taking very good care of her. Don't you worry, we are on top of it. I can see her again in my office tomorrow," he concluded.

I tried a rebuttal.

"I have no doubt that they are a good family, and it sounds like you're doing everything that needs to be done for her cancer," I started, "but I don't know if I feel totally comfortable performing a procedure on a patient for a problem that they do not even know that they have. I feel like if I'm going to stick a needle in her, then at least she should know why, no?"

"Yes, yes, it's a problem, I understand. If you don't feel comfortable then we can just do it tomorrow. She is uncomfortable but it's not dangerous to wait another day. I can see her in my office and we can figure everything out then."

He was certainly agreeable. He even seemed to understand my concern. Yet he solved it not by addressing the thorny issue of our ethical obligation to the patient, but by finding a way to absolve me of responsibility. The issue of our patient being unaware that she had cancer remained.

I told him that I would see what I could do and thanked him for taking the time to chat.

I hung up the phone somewhat more uncomfortable than I was before. The people who knew her best, it seemed, were all in agreement. Her loved ones and her physician felt comfortable treating her without her knowledge or consent. Indeed, they had already been doing it for some time. Furthermore, they all spoke her language and shared her culture. Undoubtedly, they understood her better than I ever would.

I had yet to speak with her and could not even do so except through the assistance of a telephone interpreter. Yet it increasingly looked as if it were I alone who wanted to tell this poor lady that she had cancer. It felt bold to think that everyone close to this patient—everyone who knew her well and who cared for her—was wrong and that I was right. I second-guessed my prior moral certainty.

I gathered my thoughts and ultimately decided that, at the very least, I would have to speak directly with the patient myself in order to better understand the situation. I decided that I would talk to her to try to gain a better understanding of what *she* thought was going on. At the very least, I figured, I would be able to see how she reacted before I did anything else.

I entered the room again. Telling the patient's daughter I did not feel comfortable treating her mother without at least speaking directly with her, I began to dial for the translator. She kept a stern eye on me, but, to my surprise, she did not resist.

Holding one handset to my ear and placing the other one beside my patient's, I began. "Hello, Ms. P, I am Dr. Nahvi, one of the emergency room doctors here. I'm part of the team that's taking care of you today. Can you tell me—"

She cut me off and asked her daughter to step out of the room. I do not speak a word of Greek, but the tone was unmistakably that of a chiding mother.

"Listen, you're a young doctor. I am old but not dumb. I know what's going on. I know I have cancer but my family wants to make sure that I do not know. They think it is too much for me. It's okay, just do whatever they want you to do. My daughter can be an idiot but she's trying her best." Her tone was simultaneously stern and sweet. She held my hand as she spoke into the phone as if in kind reassurance while the translator spoke to me.

"But listen." She shifted her tone and became more serious. She continued to hold my hand as she now looked me in the eye. "Don't tell my daughter that I know about my cancer. It would make her very upset if she knew that I knew. Okay?"

As if chastised by my own mother, I nodded my head obediently.

"You're young, do you have children?" she then demanded. I shook my head no.

"See, you don't understand. You will one day but right now you don't." She paused and held my hand again before continuing. "You're very sweet. Thank you." She smiled and patted my hand as one would do to provide positive reinforcement for a child performing a good deed. We hung up the phones.

I tried to catch up with my thoughts. My immediate dilemma was resolved. I no longer had to decide how to navigate *whether* to tell her that she had cancer. Indeed, there was nothing to reveal as nothing was actually ever hidden. As the patient's daughter, her personal physician, and I disagreed about *whether* to tell her, the patient herself, it appeared, had long known about her diagnosis and had rendered pointless the entire premise of our debate.

What struck me about the episode was that even as each decision that was made appeared to be wrong or backward, the conflict seemed to work itself out in the end. Each player in the episode seemed to be making some critical error in judgment, yet, at the same time, the wheels never fell off the bus. What seemed to matter more than any individual decision was the genuine human concern and compassion behind it as it was made. Thus what kept the situation moving along without it revealing itself for the ridiculous charade that it was, was each person's genuine concern for the others.

At every stage, each actor seemed to be somewhat flexible. The only thing that was determined to be nonnegotiable was that everything be done with the right intention. It was this intention—the intention to do what they thought was best for their loved one, however misguided—that seemed to matter most in the end. I went ahead and performed the procedure on Ms. P, who was fully aware of her ovarian cancer.

As I walked with Anthony to a private room to chat once more, I wondered about my responsibility to him and to Lola.

Did my inability to inform Lola about her pregnancy prohibit me from telling Anthony about it? Or, understanding that the overwhelming odds were that she would want me to tell him, and understanding that he had a right to know the cause of his wife's death, was the information simply too important for me to hold back?

Furthermore, it felt important that Anthony was still alive while Lola, of course, was dead. Does the status of one's existence matter when considering one's obligations to them? Does one have a greater obligation to the living than to the dead?

I decided to take a cue from my Greek comedy. I knew that I would not feel completely comfortable with any decision at the end of the day. Whether I told Anthony or whether I kept the information from him, I knew that I would be left feeling uneasy. No matter what I did, I would either have to risk doing wrong by Lola, or I would have to risk doing wrong by Anthony. And so, like my Greek patient and her family, I decided that I had no choice but to trust my intentions.

Anthony finally walked out of the room and signaled that he was ready. We sat down once more.

I began. "You may have noticed the IVs we placed in Lola's arms when you arrived. When she was initially brought to us by the paramedics, we inserted the IVs to give her some of our medicines, but also in order to draw blood for blood tests in the laboratory. As the results trickled back, though, some of them were unexpected."

I paused. "You had mentioned that you two had tried to get pregnant for years but were unable to." I swallowed. "I don't know how much of a surprise this may be, but when I went through her laboratory results, Lola's pregnancy test came back positive. She was pregnant."

He said nothing.

"There's more," I continued.

"We still need confirmation about what I am about to say, so there is a chance that this may not be the case, but most likely, her pregnancy probably explains *why* all of this happened. Your wife had two days of abdominal pain that got much worse today. There's a good chance that her pregnancy was what was causing her pain all along. It's something we call an ectopic pregnancy . . ."

I went on to explain to him how it was possible that their baby had grown, ruptured Lola's fallopian tube, and caused her to bleed to death from the inside.

Many emergency room doctors and nurses develop superstitious beliefs. "It's going to be a rough night tonight," the nurses I work with sometimes tell me whenever a full moon is out. And it is not uncommon for someone to get chastised if they note aloud, while at work, that a shift is particularly quiet. It is a common belief in the emergency room that invoking the "q word" can cause the remainder of a shift to become especially busy. I once had a colleague who believed she could predict who would survive and who would die based on how decent a person the patient appeared to be. "It's better to be lucky than to be good," she would say with sincerity. "Only the good people die young. It's the assholes who live forever."

I am not superstitious. Yet, in that moment, I found myself telling Anthony that I knew that Lola was a good person.

SEVENTEEN

"WHAT IS THE CRAZIEST THING YOU'VE SEEN IN THE ER?"

Finally, the time felt right to stand up and walk out of that room. I did so quietly, without interrupting to say goodbye, and closed the door behind me as I exited.

My shift had officially ended long ago and the daytime physician had already arrived. I was no longer required to remain in the emergency room so I decided to step outside to clear my head. I stood in the cold for several minutes, thinking about nothing in particular as I watched my humid breath hit the winter air. It was a clear morning and the dawn sunlight reflected off the hospital's windows. A handful of chirping birds gathered in the courtyard of a nearby church. Despite whatever I was experiencing inside the hospital, outside, life continued on normally.

It felt strange that such intensity could be so rigidly confined. The energy in the emergency room often makes it feel as if the entire world should be on edge. I recall one shift where patients were arriving at such a fast pace and with such severity of disease that I actually paused to check the news. Surely some big and catastrophic event must have occurred, I thought.

Of course, hurricanes and terrorist explosions do not cause patients to develop bowel ischemia or ruptured aortic aneurysms. I loaded the news only to find the usual headlines. There was no bold typeface. Both inside and outside the emergency room, it was a regular day.

Across the street, an old man strolled by, walking his old beagle behind him. The old dog stopped every few steps, making sure to investigate whatever it was they came across. Potted plants, berried bushes, and torn trash bags leaking mystery fluids were all of equal interest. I appreciated the dog's instinct—nothing was too common, too boring, or too off-putting to walk past and ignore. The old man refused to rush his dog, allowing him to explore his world as he saw fit. They seemed to share an understanding.

There was something cathartic about watching the geriatric pair. Unhurried and guided only by their whims and impulses, they were engaged in the critical task of simply enjoying their moment. They seemed to exude a sort of wisdom.

I exhaled and watched one more breath blend into the air before making my way back inside to wrap up my remaining tasks, including one last bureaucratic demand. After filling out Lola's online paperwork, I had to speak with the medical examiner over the phone. After every death, it is our job to call the Office of the Chief Medical Examiner to discuss the case. Together, we decide whether or not an autopsy is performed.

The medical examiner, of course, does not exist to simply

solve the mystery of a death. Employed by the city and tasked with the public interest in mind, the Office of the Chief Medical Examiner investigates death primarily to safeguard against it. Medical examiners dissect human bodies to search for clues. They identify inflammatory tissue, they biopsy disease, and they pinpoint bullet trajectories. They share their findings with other government agencies like the health department, the poison control center, and the police department. As a result of their work, close contacts of someone who died of meningitis might be prescribed a course of prophylactic antibiotics, a school might have its water supply sterilized after the identification of a nearby outbreak of legionella, and a murder suspect might be apprehended before he can go on to commit further harm.

For this reason, the medical examiner will generally accept for autopsy any patient who dies despite being young and healthy, any patient who dies under suspicious circumstances, or any patient who dies as the result of violent means. These cases contain the most potential to provide clues, uncover answers, and save lives. Most other deaths, however—the vast majority of deaths that take place, in fact—are not sent to the medical examiner. These bodies go to the morgue for storage until a funeral can be arranged or until it is clear that nobody will be coming forward to claim the body. We may ultimately be unsure whether a patient has died of a heart attack, stroke, or an asthma exacerbation, for example, but in the absence of a particular reason to look into it, we usually do not take the steps to find out.[1]

Early in my career, I was struck by how few cases were actually accepted by the medical examiner. I may have known nothing about my patient except that they were elderly, had a medical history of diabetes and high blood pressure, and that they were now dead—yet that was often enough. "Okay, that makes sense," the medical examiner would comment over the phone, finding the death of my patient to be reasonable enough based on nothing more than the casual knowledge that old people with high blood pressure and diabetes sometimes die.

Before entering medicine, I had always assumed that our systems were more sophisticated than I found them to be. If a car mechanic can use computerized diagnostics to determine the precise reason a "check engine" light came on, I thought surely our medical system has a comparable set of tools to identify the malfunctions of a human body. The truth, however, is that so much of medicine is vague and imprecise. We might be able to track a pizza we order on the internet from the moment it exits the oven to the instant it is delivered to our door, but we often cannot tell family members what precisely caused their loved one to die.

I called the medical examiner, read off Lola's demographics, and provided a brief summary of her circumstance. "Oh wow, that sounds interesting," she responded. Coming from someone who deals exclusively with curious and violent deaths, it was a striking acknowledgment. Because Lola was young and because the likely cause of her death was somewhat rare, the medical examiner would accept the case.

I went back to the room where Lola was lying. I had to inform the nursing team of the medical examiner's decision. When no autopsy is requested by the medical examiner, every tube, IV line, and miscellaneous piece of tape must be removed so that the body can be sent to the morgue and then a funeral home. Appearance, not answers, is what is important in these circumstances. When an autopsy is requested, on the other hand, everything is to remain in place. The city uses everything it can to search for hints and clues in an attempt to identify a cause of death.

I took another look at Lola. Her body was now covered with white sheets. Her skin had developed a somewhat purple hue. Although she was colder and more swollen, without the excitement of the resuscitation I was finally able to see her more clearly.

I noticed her hands. They had a fresh coat of nail polish. I wondered if she had recently gotten a manicure.

One can become accustomed to gunshot wounds, stabbings, or grotesquely deforming head traumas. These injuries, no matter how unsightly, point to how the patient died. Recent manicures and fresh haircuts, on the other hand, are much more striking. Much like a family photo one might find in a patient's wallet, they are signs of life. They force one to think not about how that patient died, but how they lived.

A patient I cared for years earlier had worked for the city in the Department of Sanitation when he died while on shift. His coworkers called an ambulance and escorted him to the emergency room. While the details surrounding his medical care have blurred with time, the particulars of a tattoo he had have stayed with me. In the midst of our efforts to resuscitate him, I remember observing a large saber-tooth tiger snarling at nothing in particular over the right side of his chest. It was still covered in cellophane wrap, indicating he had it completed only recently. It felt strange to note the brand-new tattoo on his dead body. *Tattoos are permanent*, I remember thinking—most people who get them probably expect them to last for decades. Rare is the tattoo that only lasts a couple of days. And so, in this way, despite being face to face with his actual death, it was this patient's tattoo that truly captured life's fragility.

I mentioned Lola's manicured hands to Alexandria, the young but motherly nurse.

"Oh wow, they're beautiful," she said with sincerity as Lola's hands dangled.

I was not quite sure what to make of her answer—but then again, I was not quite sure what to make of my remark, either. Despite confronting the extraordinary, it is always the everyday things that hold our attention.

After finding out what I do for a living, in addition to asking me how I deal with the stress of working in the emergency room people also like to routinely ask, "What is the craziest thing you've seen in the ER?" I imagine they want to hear the types of stories that might be aired on a television show set in an emergency room. I usually offer them another story of retrieving an object from a patient's rectum or one of the more dramatic successes our trauma surgeons might have had.

That said, those stories rarely interest me. The most honest answer I might be able to give to this question also happens to be the most pedestrian. Grocery lists, coffee shop rewards cards, new tattoos, and fresh manicures—these are the things that really reflect the full extent of our experiences.

I decided that the next time I was asked the question, I would answer, "Grocery lists and tattoos. Trust me, they can be wild."

EIGHTEEN

THE LOTTO TICKET

Having handed off my active patients to the daytime doctor, I wrapped up any loose ends that remained. The sun rose higher into the winter sky, reminding me how far past the end of my shift I had lingered. Finally, I was ready to leave. I went to the locker room and changed out of my scrubs and into my street clothes.

I checked in with Daniela."Thanks for your help tonight. I know there was a lot going on—do you have any questions about anything we did?" She shook her head no and gave me a confident smile. I couldn't help but think of all the times throughout my training where my mind staggered with thoughts while I made sure to project an air of casual self-assuredness.

I searched for Anthony one last time. I found him back in his wife's room. Two other men were now with him—he had called his family, or perhaps some friends, to join him. I gave them a cautious smile. The number of people who are forced to deal with death alone is disheartening. I was happy he had some support. I walked over to say goodbye and to tell him that I was heading home.

For the briefest of moments, he looked at me puzzled. My change of clothes must have caught him off guard. Patients often fail to recognize us when we are not in our white coats or scrubs.

On more than one occasion, after an extended interaction with a patient over the course of many hours in the emergency room, I have waved to them on the sidewalk as we both made our way home. Often, they failed to recognize me until they squinted their eyes, and then, moments later, waved back. This type of situation has occurred enough times that I no longer doubt Clark Kent's disguise of nothing more than a change of clothes and a pair of glasses.

Just as I gain a greater appreciation for my patients as I learn more about them, however, I imagine these brief interactions might provide our patients a better understanding of us.

I remember once, as a child, seeing my second-grade teacher in the supermarket. I remember feeling startled at seeing her there. I must have assumed that she lived in the school—that she ate her dinners in the cafeteria and that she would roll out a sleeping bag in the gymnasium when it was time to go to bed. Seeing her outside of the usual context I was accustomed to seeing her in, I was forced to understand her in a new light.

I asked Anthony if there was anything else he needed. He shook his head and thanked me once again. I lowered my head in sympathy and waved as I walked away. It was an awkward end to a long night, but there was no good way for me to have left him.

I said a quick goodbye to Alexandria, Daris, Danny, and the others who worked so hard alongside me and who shared the night's experience. I was lucky to work with such a wonderful group.

Alexandria smiled and waved and Daris saluted. "See you for round two later today!" Danny yelled with a chuckle. He was technically right. I would be seeing them all later that same day. When you work the overnight shift, work schedules become unsynchronized with the calendar. We were walking out of the hospital on a Wednesday morning, and would be seeing each other again on Wednesday evening. Even when we sleep after an overnight shift, because we wake up in the same day we went to sleep in, we don't have that sense of a reset upon waking back up. It is difficult to put yesterday's shift behind you when yesterday's shift is still today.

"See you later today, Danny," I said and smiled.

Finally, I stepped through the automatic doors that opened into the ambulance bay. I saw Winston and Lewis parked in their ambulance just outside.

"What ended up happening with that last lady we brought in?" they asked. "She was pretty young, no?"

"Nothing really changed after you guys left—she stayed dead." I gave an uncertain shrug. "Turns out she was pregnant, though. Looks like it must have been an ectopic."

"Wow, that's wild. Get home safe, man."

"Yeah, totally crazy, right? Thanks for all your help. See you guys tonight."

My fingers complained about the cold air, but the warmth of the sun soothed my face. I put on my helmet and head-phones, unchained my bicycle, and hopped on.

As I glided through the streets on my bicycle, my racing thoughts evaporated. On a deeper level, however, every pa-tient encounter remains with you. Each one adds a new flavor, texture, and richness to life and our understanding of it.

I sped through a red light. A driver honked his horn and cursed me from his window. I smiled back. I huffed as I rode across the interborough bridge. I decided to take the long route home through the park. Children were playing on the playground and dogs were being walked off leash in the early morning hour.

As I neared my apartment, the corner of my eye caught the flashing New York Lottery sign by the bodega on the corner. I do not play the lotto but I gravitated toward it today.

I paid a dollar at the register and the attendant handed me the ticket. "Good luck," he said as I walked out the door.

I smiled.

Don't you realize? I thought to myself, *we've both already won.*

EPILOGUE

After the final no there comes a yes,
And on that yes the future world depends.

      —Wallace Stevens, "The Well Dressed Man with a Beard"

I once cared for a patient who had arrived at my emergency room complaining of some chest pain. She was a young woman in her forties, she had no comorbid medical problems, and her description of the pain was not typical for a heart attack, a blood clot, or any other dangerous diagnosis that a complaint of chest pain might represent. In short, I did not believe she was suffering from any serious disease.

Nevertheless, in the emergency room we take claims of chest pain seriously. All of us who work there have had at least one experience with a patient who suffered a heart attack despite our textbooks telling us they had no right to do so. So, in order to ensure that the facts supported my instinct, I conducted a brief medical workup consisting of an EKG, a chest x-ray, and some basic blood tests. These tests all returned with normal results.

I recall informing this patient of her normal results,

reassuring her that her heart and lungs appeared healthy, and telling her that she was safe to return home. She nodded her head in understanding and prepared to depart, before hesitating and turning back to me.

"I can't, I just can't," she said with a sense of urgency.

"You can't what?" I asked.

"I can't go back." She started sobbing.

"You can't go back where?" I followed up.

"I can't go back to *that*. I can't do it, I just can't do it," she replied, now bawling and having worked herself up to an emotional pitch.

Worried that she was suffering from domestic violence, suicidality, or some other hidden danger, I questioned her about the specific threat she was facing. She dismissed my attempts, insisting that she was not in any immediate harm. The "that" that so terrified her was simply her day-to-day existence. She told me that she was a single mother working as a housekeeper to provide for her two children. "I work and I work and I work seven days a week and I never stop and if I stop we have nothing. My bosses are so cruel and they push me and push me but I need to work so what can I do? This is not life. This is torture." She sat back down on the hospital gurney and cried into my shoulder.

I remained silent. I did not know what to say. When I did speak, I could only think to offer her expressions of sympathy and the resources we have to offer from the emergency room: the evaluation of a psychiatrist, a phone call to the police so that she could file a report if she felt a crime had been committed, a conversation with our social worker to see if she was eligible for any social services. She refused all of these. With an emergency room overrun with ill and injured patients who had each been waiting hours to be seen, I could not even offer her the resource of my time: I could not just sit down with her to have a long conversation. Ultimately she regained her composure and apologized for her display of humanity. "I'm sorry, I know there's nothing you could do about any of this, it's not your problem." She stood up and wiped her eyes. "I'll be okay," she reassured me as she walked toward the exit.

Another time, I cared for a young woman after a suicide attempt. She was the victim of a sex trafficker and had been brought to New York from her home country in Central America. In order to prevent her from going to the police, her traffickers made threats against her family. She attempted to escape her circumstance not by running to the authorities, but by drinking from a container of household bleach. That she survived, I believe, was only because of a lack of information. Unlike the industrial variety, household bleach is usually not strong enough to cause any serious damage, even with ingestion. I have no doubt that, had she been aware of this critical bit of information, she would have been dead.

Upon hearing her story, I was not only troubled, but was once again left wondering what I could do to help. After all, her ultimate problem was not medical. She had no chemical imbalance in her brain that caused her to feel depressed and harm herself. There was no organic disturbance of her body's hormones. She was, in fact, responding understandably to a life circumstance so horrendous that it was difficult to even imagine its depths. Her suicide attempt did not reflect something wrong with her, but something wrong with the world around her.

Without any other available options, however, and knowing that simply discharging her home would have been catastrophic, we admitted her to the psychiatric floors, as we do all patients who have survived a suicide attempt. There she was given antidepressant medications and was stripped of any firm or sharp objects that could have been used for any further attempts at self-harm.

These sorts of interactions are not uncommon in a modern emergency room. Yet they leave us with a particular sense of unease. As in my interaction with Lola and Anthony and in so many of the other stories shared in this book, it is the uneasiness of being up close with the rawest form of the human condition, only to have to walk away with no real resolution and no clean sense of closure.

This book is my response to so many of these moments of unease.

Over and over again during my years of working in the emergency room, I would find myself walking away from an interaction with a patient or their family member only to feel this very particular sense of unease. It was often accompanied by an exasperated confusion that left me wondering, *What now? This experience was clearly important, but what do I do with it? What lesson could I possibly draw from it and how does it fit into my understanding of the world?*

I found it difficult to let these experiences go. I would bring them home with me, then back to work the next day, and then home again. I would dwell on them and spend many restless nights troubled by them. On walks with my dog, on bicycle rides crossing the boroughs, and at social gatherings where others were present but I was somehow not, I found myself trying to wrap my head around these questions and, somehow, answer them.

Because these were questions for which no answers exist, of course, I could not. Ultimately, I came to appreciate that my approach was shortsighted. If I was going to make sense of anything, I realized, I would have to reframe my questions and, with them, my entire perspective. And so, "How might these experiences make sense given my understanding of the world?" eventually turned into, "What *is* my understanding of the world given the truth of these experiences?"

For me then, in this way, the ideas and themes explored in this book were simply a starting point for something greater. I hope that they can be the same for you. I hope that my unsolved dilemmas and unanswered questions can provide you with a measure of discomfort. I hope that this discomfort can stir you to consider some of life's most important questions—questions that are tremendously important, but that we often find so easy to ignore. Whatever journey these questions may lead you on and whatever conclusions you may come to, I hope that you too can learn to appreciate our uncomfortable experiences, welcome their nuance and subtlety, and come to enjoy their uncertainty.

Life is raw, it is fragile, and it is beautiful. Often, it is discomfiting. When we find that it is, we should treat these discomfiting bits of life in much the same way we treat a sculpture in a museum. We should inspect it and take the time to walk around it, analyzing it from every angle and appreciating the way every ray of light bounces off each of its different surfaces. We might find that what may look ordinary from one perspective may be extraordinary from another.

Our everyday lives are meaningful and profound. It is worth slowing down to take a closer look.

Acknowledgments

On page 54, the line, "that verdict was already made, and even the best that medicine had to offer could make no appeal," is inspired by a sentence from the book *Wind, Sand, and Stars*, by Antoine de Saint-Exupéry ("Fate has pronounced a decision from which there is no appeal"). As I worked through the ideas that became the foundation of this book, I was guided by the writings of Saint-Exupéry and the poems of the fourteenth-century Persian poet Hafez. From different eras, continents, and cultures, these writers share a love of life and a clear vision of what makes life worth living—I consider them not only inspirations, but friends.

I would also like to thank a few people, in no particular order, who made this work possible.

To my patients, for allowing me the opportunity to engage in the most human act of caring for one another. Thank you for teaching me so much about life. To the nurses, PAs, clerks, scribes, custodial staff, respiratory therapists, patient technicians, residents, medical students, and so many others I get to work alongside. Thank you for being there with me and thank you for being there for me.

ACKNOWLEDGMENTS

To my agent, Alice Martell, for your enthusiasm for this book and for your confidence in me from the very beginning. To my editor, Bob Bender, for your patience and for clearly understanding what I was trying to accomplish with this book even at its earliest stages. Thank you both for your tireless work and for placing your trust in me as a writer.

To my sister, Barin, for being not only this book's first editor but also my life editor. Thank you for enduring the early drafts of this book and for supporting it nonetheless, and thank you for enduring the early drafts of me and supporting me nonetheless. To my wife, Vivian, for our love collaboration. Thank you for listening to my endless attempts at trying to make sense of what is senseless, and thank you for letting me spend my life with you. To Aghdass and Mehdi, my mother and father, for leading by the example of your values and for your inexhaustible and unconditional love. This book would not exist, and neither would I, without all of you.

To Dr. Lewis Goldfrank, Dr. Anand Swaminathan, and Dr. Inna Leybell for being my mentors and for reading this book in its earliest manuscript phase. Thank you for teaching me how to practice emergency medicine, and more importantly, thank you for showing me not only what it means to be a skilled doctor, but a good one.

To my peers whose text message exchanges appear in the prologue of this book. Thank you for being the brilliant and talented people you are, and thank you for letting me learn with you and from you over the past decade.

To the New York Public Library, for providing a space in which much of this book was written.

ACKNOWLEDGMENTS

To the rappers and artists who inspired in me a love of language: Jay-Z, Himanshu Suri, Riz Ahmed, Killer Mike, Starlito, Sean Price, Ms. Lauryn Hill and the Fugees, Boots Riley and the Coup, Mos Def, the Wu-Tang Clan, A Tribe Called Quest, dead prez, Talib Kweli, The Notorious B.I.G., Outkast, Common, Earthgang, MF Doom, Del the Funky Homosapien, Prince Paul and Dan the Automator, the Beastie Boys, Cody ChesnuTT, David Bowie, Johnny Cash, Lin-Manuel Miranda, Leonard Cohen, and so many others. Thank you for showing me the power of painting pictures with words.

Notes

Prologue. The Novel Coronavirus

1. Breathing serves two functions: supplying the body with oxygen and eliminating carbon dioxide from the lungs. Respiratory failure occurs when either of these two functions has failed. In this case, the patient experienced hypoxic respiratory failure, indicating a failure of oxygen delivery.

2. Nasal cannula and a nonrebreather facemask are two modalities for providing oxygen to patients. A nonrebreather mask can provide higher concentrations of oxygen than a nasal cannula. It is an escalation in therapy. To "tube" someone is to intubate them. It is the most aggressive form of respiratory support.

3. "Vents" refers to ventilators.

4. S. M. Lim, W. C. Cha, M. K. Chae, and I. J. Jo, "Contamination during doffing of personal protective equipment by healthcare providers," *Clinical and Experimental Emergency Medicine,* 2(3) (2015): 162–67; doi: 10.15441/ceem.15.019; PMID: 27752591; PMCID: PMC5052842.

5. H. Kanamori, D. J. Weber, and W. A. Rutala, "The role of the healthcare surface environment in SARS-CoV-2 transmission and potential control measures," *Clinical Infectious Diseases,* September 28, 2020; ciaa1467; doi: 10.1093/cid/ciaa1467; e-pub ahead of print; PMID: 32985671; PMCID: PMC7543309.

6. A high-flow nasal cannula is yet another modality for delivering oxygen to patients. It provides higher concentrations of oxygen than a regular nasal cannula or a nonrebreather mask, but less support than a ventilator.

7. This colleague suffered respiratory failure not from a failure of breathing's first function (supplying oxygen to the body) but from its second, the elimination of carbon dioxide. This occurred because her lungs were not ventilating (inflating and deflating) properly, causing carbon dioxide to become "retained" in her body, which in turn caused her blood to become acidic. In order to ensure that this sequence of events would not threaten the fetus that shared her blood, the doctors caring for her decided to perform a Caesarean section and deliver her baby while she remained in a medically induced coma.

8. Statistical power is used in research to determine how likely it is that a study has distinguished an actual effect from one that might have been observed by chance. It is usually a consequence of how large a study's sample size is.

9. N. van Doremalen et al., "Aerosol and Surface Stability of SARS-CoV-2 as Compared with SARS-CoV-1," *New England Journal of Medicine,* 382(16) (2020): 1564–67; doi: 10.1056/NEJMc2004973; e-pub March 17, 2020; PMID: 32182409; PMCID: PMC7121658.

10. "Treated Like Trash: Mt. Sinai Nurses Wearing Garbage Bags as Coronavirus Supplies Dry," *New York Post,* March 26, 2020, cover page.

11. Somini Sengupta, "A N.Y. Nurse Dies. Angry Co-Workers Blame a Lack of Protective Gear," *New York Times,* March 26, 2020.

12. Kenneth G. Langone, Robert I. Grossman, Steven B. Abramson, Robert J. Cerfolio, Fritz François, Joseph Greco, and Bret J. Rudy, Letter to the Editor: "NYU Must Compensate Its Medical Workers Fairly," *Washington Square News,* April 20, 2020.

NOTES

13. Emily Baumgaertner, "COVID-19 doctors running out of masks? Try a bandanna, the CDC says," *Los Angeles Times,* March 21, 2020.

14. K. A. Hill et al., "Assessment of the Prevalence of Medical Student Mistreatment by Sex, Race/Ethnicity, and Sexual Orientation," *JAMA Internal Medicine,* 180(5) (2020): 653–65; doi: 10.1001/jamainternmed.2020.0030; PMID: 32091540; PMCID: PMC7042809.

15. Matt Richtel, "At the Hospital, a Face-Off Over Face Masks," *New York Times,* April 7, 2020, Section D, Page 7.

16. Akela Lacy, "Kaiser Permanente Threatened to Fire Nurses Treating Covid-19 Patients for Wearing Their Own Masks, Unions Say," *Intercept,* March 24, 2020.

17. Ashley Hiruko, "This Anesthesiologist Was Told to Not Wear a Face Mask Amid COVID-19 Crisis," KUOW, Puget Sound Public Radio, March 27, 2020.

18. Leila Fadel, "Doctors Say Hospitals Are Stopping Them from Wearing Masks," National Public Radio, April 2, 2020, special series: *The Coronavirus Crisis.*

19. Nicholas Kristof, "We're Betraying Our Doctors and Nurses," *New York Times,* April 2, 2020, Section A, Page 24.

20. Testing was also available for those who had directly returned from a handful of countries including China, South Korea, Iran, Macau, and several others.

21. Fentanyl is an opioid medication used for pain control.

22. Propofol is a medication used to sedate patients. It is often used for patients who are intubated.

23. "Pumps" refers to infusion pumps. These are the machines that attach to intravenous lines and allow for the calibrated delivery of medications into a patient's veins.

24. "Azithro" refers to azithromycin. It is an antibiotic often used to treat bacterial pneumonias.

25. "Portable vents" refers to portable ventilators. These are small, mobile ventilators that are battery powered and often lack the full feature set of an intensive care unit ventilator. In normal circumstances, they are used for short periods of time and reserved for instances where the use of a full-sized ventilator would not be possible, such as when transporting patients in a hospital's elevators.

26. Ayesha Rascoe, "Trump Resists Using Wartime Law to Get, Distribute Coronavirus Supplies," *Morning Edition,* National Public Radio, March 25, 2020.

27. Zeynep Tufekci, "Why Did It Take So Long to Accept the Facts About Covid?" *New York Times,* May 7, 2021.

28. Lena Sun, "Face Mask Shortage Prompts CDC to Loosen Coronavirus Guidance," *Washington Post,* March 10, 2020.

29. Zeynep Tufekci, "Why Did It Take So Long to Accept the Facts About Covid?" *New York Times,* May 7, 2021.

30. Jane Spencer and Christina Jewett, "12 Months of Trauma: More Than 3,600 US Health Workers Died in Covid's First Year," *Kaiser Health News,* April 8, 2021.

31. J. Y. Choi, "COVID-19 in South Korea," *Postgraduate Medical Journal,* 96(1137) (2020): 399–402; doi: 10.1136/postgrad medj-2020-137738; e-pub May 4, 2020; PMID: 32366457.

32. Michael Sullivan, "In Vietnam, There Have Been Fewer Than 300 COVID-19 Cases and No Deaths. Here's Why," National Public Radio, April 16, 2020.

33. L. Morawska and D. K. Milton, "It Is Time to Address Airborne Transmission of Coronavirus Disease 2019 (COVID-19)," *Clinical Infectious Diseases,* 71(9) (2020): 2311–313; doi: 10.1093/cid/ciaa939; PMID: 32628269; PMCID: PMC7454469.

34. Amelia Wade, "Prime Minister Jacinda Ardern on Govt's extra millions on PPE," *New Zealand Herald,* June 28, 2020.

35. Mario Parker and Josh Wingrove, "Trump Suggests a New York Hospital Is Losing Masks Because of Crime," *Bloomberg News,* March 29, 2020.

36. Jemima McEvoy, "'We've Done Worse Than Most Any Other Country': Fauci Says 500,000 Covid-19 Deaths Didn't Need to Happen," *Forbes,* February 22, 2021.

37. Lisa Schnirring, "CDC unveils new PPE guidance for Ebola," *CIDRAP News,* Center for Infectious Disease Research and Policy, University of Minnesota, October 20, 2014.

38. R. M. Ratwani, A. Fong, J. S. Puthumana, and A. Z. Hettinger, "Emergency Physician Use of Cognitive Strategies to Manage Interruptions," *Annals of Emergency Medicine,* 70(5) (2017): 683–87; doi: 10.1016/j.annemergmed.2017.04.036; PMID: 28601266.

39. A noninvasive ventilator is a ventilator that employs an external facemask (rather than a tube inserted in the mouth) to assist patients' breathing.

40. P. Chen et al., "SARS-CoV-2 Neutralizing Antibody LY-CoV555 in Outpatients with Covid-19," *New England Journal of Medicine,* 384(3) (2021): 229–37; doi: 10.1056/NEJMoa2029849; e-pub October 28, 2020; PMID: 33113295; PMCID: PMC7646625.

41. D. M. Weinreich et al., "REGN-COV2, a Neutralizing Antibody Cocktail, in Outpatients with Covid-19," *New England Journal of Medicine,* 384(3) (2021): 238–51; doi: 10.1056/NEJMoa2035002; e-pub December 17, 2020; PMID: 33332778; PMCID: PMC7781102.

42. Evidence from before the pandemic demonstrated that about half of all emergency room doctors suffer from clinical burnout, causing many of them to leave the workforce early. Evidence from before the pandemic also demonstrated that physicians suffer from depression and suicide at twice the rates of the general population. Many predict that the Covid-19 pandemic will be followed by a second-wave crisis among healthcare workers. While this may be true, the greater truth is that we have already been living that crisis for years. See:

C. R. Stehman, Z. Testo, R. S. Gershaw, and A. R. Kellogg,

"Burnout, Drop Out, Suicide: Physician Loss in Emergency Medicine, Part I," *Western Journal of Emergency Medicine,* 20(3) (2019): 485–94; doi: 10.5811/westjem.2019.4.40970; e-pub April 23, 2019; errata in, *Western Journal of Emergency Medicine,* 20(5) (2019): 840–41; PMID: 31123550; PMCID: PMC6526882.

Q. Zhang, M. C. Mu, Y. He, Z. L. Cai, and Z. C. Li, "Burnout in emergency medicine physicians: A meta-analysis and systematic review," *Medicine* (Baltimore), 99(32) (2020): e21462; doi: 10.1097/MD.0000000000021462; PMID: 32769876; PMCID: PMC7593073.

A. Boutou, G. Pitsiou, E. Sourla, and I. Kioumis, "Burnout syndrome among emergency medicine physicians: An update on its prevalence and risk factors," *European Review for Medical and Pharmacological Sciences,* 23(20) (2019): 9058–65; doi: 10.26355/eurrev_201910_19308. PMID: 31696496.

Pauline Anderson, "Physicians Experience Highest Suicide Rate of Any Profession," *Medscape Medical News,* May 7, 2018.

Blake Farmer, "When Doctors Struggle with Suicide, Their Profession Often Fails Them," *Morning Edition,* National Public Radio, July 31, 2018.

One. Death's Herald

1. "Walkie-talkie": Medical jargon for "walking and talking," it is a shorthand way to communicate that the patient is capable of these basic life functions, indicating that they are not in extremis (a patient with a severe breathing issue, for example, often cannot talk, and a patient with a severe neurological issue like a stroke, for example, often cannot walk). "Antecube" is short for antecubital fossa. This is the soft side of the elbow where large and easily accessible veins are often found. Asystole is a cardiac rhythm in which the heart has ceased any electrical or mechanical activity. "Epi" is short for epinephrine, a medication

with many purposes that is routinely used in resuscitation efforts in patients who have died.

2. GlideScope is a brand of fiber optic video laryngoscope, used to visualize a patient's airway when performing an intubation. "ET tube" is short for endotracheal tube. This is the name for the actual plastic tube that is placed in a patient's trachea and connected to a ventilator.

3. Glucose, or blood sugar, is always checked immediately upon encountering a dead patient. Glucose levels that are either too high or too low are two of the few correctable, reversible causes of death.

Four. The Orchestra and Its Audience of One

1. Danny was one of the members of our team who, during our Covid-19 crisis, would have a brush with death himself. Suffering respiratory failure, he was intubated in the intensive care unit at a time when the predicted mortality rate was estimated to be around 85 percent for such an event. His eventual recovery was a cause for celebration.

2. Whereas an IV refers to an intravenous line, an IO refers to an intraosseous line, or a tube that is drilled directly into a patient's bone. While an IO is a somewhat more aggressive procedure, both an IV and an IO are equally effective at administering blood, fluids, or medications. An IO line is often used in critical settings when an intravenous line cannot be rapidly obtained.

Five. A Desperate Search for Clues

1. The research I refer to in this chapter includes: P. Jabre et al., "Family presence during cardiopulmonary resuscitation," *New England Journal of Medicine,* 368(11) (2013): 1008–18; doi: 10.1056/NEJMoa1203366; PMID: 23484827. C. De Stefano et al., "Family Presence during Resuscitation: A Qualitative Analysis from a National Multicenter Randomized Clinical Trial," *PLoS One,* 11(6) (2016): e0156100; doi: 10.1371/journal.pone.0156100;

NOTES

PMID: 27253993; PMCID: PMC4890739. P. Jabre et al., "Offering the opportunity for family to be present during cardiopulmonary resuscitation: 1-year assessment," *Intensive Care Medicine,* 40(7) (2014): 981–87; doi: 10.1007/s00134-014-3337-1. e-pub May 23, 2014; PMID: 24852952.

2. As a resuscitation progresses, a major part of the care team's job is to look for any potential reversible causes of death, known as the five H's (Hypovolemia, Hypoxia, Hydrogen ions, Hyper- or Hypokalemia, and Hypothermia) and five T's (these are: cardiac Tamponade, Toxins, pulmonary Thrombosis, coronary Thrombosis, and Tension pneumothorax). Illness, drug use, an actual or possible pregnancy and a personal history of blood clots can all provide important clues to help us identify a potential "H" or "T."

Six. To Recalibrate a Human Being

1. CO_2 is a normal byproduct of the body's cellular metabolism. We measure CO_2 during resuscitations, then, to determine whether the body's cells are still functioning. When we cannot measure adequate CO_2 levels, we understand that the body has died at a cellular level. ECHO refers to an echocardiogram, or a bedside ultrasound of the heart that serves as a visual adjunct to feeling for a pulse. It can help diagnose several of the reversible causes of death. The mention of glucose refers to hypo- or hyperglycemia (low or high glucose levels), one of the five H's. "Potassium issues" refers to hypo- or hyperkalemia (low or high potassium levels), another of the five H's. Hypoxia, or low oxygen levels, refers to a third "H."

2. ACS refers to acute coronary syndrome. It is the umbrella term under which a heart attack falls and is often interchangeable for coronary thrombosis, one of the five T's.

3. A pulmonary embolism is also known as a pulmonary thrombosis, another of the T's.

NOTES

Nine. Even Our Principles Stumble

1. The Emergency Medical Treatment and Active Labor Act of 1986 mandates that all patients who request care in an emergency room receive a medical screening exam and stabilization of their condition regardless of insurance status or ability to pay. This law only applies to care received in the emergency room and labor and delivery floor and does not apply to patients seeking care in other areas of the hospital, in private medical offices or clinics, or in other facilities like cancer centers or rehabilitation facilities.

2. Notably, this standard applies only to adult patients. While most children could pass this standard, these rules do not apply to them.

Eleven. The Cough That Was Cancer

1. M. W. Rabow and S. J. McPhee, "Beyond breaking bad news: How to help patients who suffer," *Western Journal of Medicine,* 171(4) (1999): 260–63; PMID: 10578682; PMCID: PMC1305864.

2. G. K. Vandekieft, "Breaking bad news," *American Family Physician,* 64(12) (2001): 1975–78; PMID: 11775763.

Thirteen. The Absurdity of Bureaucrats

1. Emergency Medicine Practice Committee, American College of Emergency Physicians, "Emergency Department Crowding: High Impact Solutions," May 2016, https://www.acep.org/globalassets/sites/acep/media/crowding/empc_crowding-ip_092016.pdf, retrieved May 14, 2021.

2. A. J. Singer, H. C. Thode, Jr., P. Viccellio, and J. M. Pines, "The association between length of emergency department boarding and mortality," *Academic Emergency Medicine,* 18(12) (2011): 1324–29; doi: 10.1111/j.1553-2712.2011.01236.x; PMID: 22168198.

3. B. C. Sun et al., "Effect of emergency department crowding on outcomes of admitted patients," *Annals of Emergency Medicine,* 61(6) (2013): 605–11.e6; doi: 10.1016/j.annemergmed.2012.10.026; e-pub December 6, 2012; PMID: 23218508; PMCID: PMC 3690784.

Fourteen. Cause of Death: ?

1. In fairness, in the time since I completed Lola's death certificate with the Office of the Chief Medical Examiner, New York's database has indeed been thoroughly revamped. Now it is app-based and uses facial recognition technology. It is, in fact, decidedly modern.

Fifteen. Knowledge Is Power. Ignorance Is Bliss

1. Martin Keith, "Medscape Internist Compensation Report 2021," Medscape, May 14, 2021.

2. Blood glucose is checked to ensure that a patient with extremely high or extremely low blood sugars is not mistaken for being intoxicated. Very high and very low blood sugars can cause one to slur their speech, slow their mental state, and appear drunk.

3. Many drunk patients sustain head injuries that can go unnoticed in their intoxicated state, so we check all of our drunk patients for any recent signs of head trauma. Furthermore, head trauma, like high or low blood glucose levels, can itself mimic the effects of intoxication. A patient who has been struck in the head and appears unusually sleepy may be assumed to be drunk when, in fact, she is suffering from life-threatening bleeding by her brain. Thus we check all of our drunk patients for signs of head trauma both to make sure that they have not unwittingly struck their heads in their drunken state, and to ensure that they are not a severely injured patient who was misunderstood to be drunk.

NOTES

Seventeen. "What Is the Craziest Thing You've Seen in the ER?"

1. If a case is rejected for autopsy by the medical examiner, family members can request a private autopsy to be performed at their own expense. A private autopsy is generally not covered by health insurance and can cost between $2,000 and $5,000. Such autopsies are rarely performed.